Inner Journey

Learning to live
with bipolar disorder

www.jamiebeggs.com.au

The National Library of Australia Cataloguing-in-Publication entry:

  Beggs, Jamie, 1968- .
  Inner journey: learning to live with bipolar.
  ISBN 0 9802945 0 9.

  1. Manic-depressive persons - Australia - Life skills
  guides. 2. Self-help techniques - Australia. I. Beggs,
  Andrew, 1966- . II. Beggs, Cameron, 1971- . III. Mintjes,
  Maaike. IV. Title.

616.895

Written by Jamie Beggs
Book Design and Production by Brown Cow Design
Produced wholly in Australia

Inner Journey

Learning to live
with bipolar disorder

Jamie Beggs

"Even a happy life cannot be without a measure of darkness and the word 'happiness' would lose its meaning if it were not balanced by sadness".

Carl Jung

What is bipolar disorder?

Bipolar (mood) disorder used to be called manic depressive illness. The new name better describes the extreme mood swings - the highs and lows - that people with this illness suffer. People with bipolar mood disorder experience recurrent episodes of depressed and elated moods, which can range from mild to severe.

'Mania' or 'hypomania' is used to describe the states of extreme elation and overactivity. Common symptoms include:

- Feeling extremely high, happy and full of energy
- Reduced need to sleep
- Irritability – the person may get irritable with people who dismiss or do not agree with unrealistic plans or ideas
- Rapid thinking ('racing thoughts') and rapid speech
- Lack of inhibitions and a lack of insight – a person experiencing mania might notice other people question his/her behaviour but is unlikely to recognise that his/her behaviour is inappropriate
- Creativity
- Mystical experiences (seeing special connections between events, believing things have a special significance)

Some people may suffer psychotic symptoms during manic episodes. They may experience grandiose or persecutory delusions, or visual, auditory, tactile or other types of hallucinations.

At the other extreme of mania is depression. People lose interest and pleasure in activities they normally enjoy. They may become withdrawn and feel even simple tasks are too demanding. They are overwhelmed by a deep sadness, find it hard to concentrate and may experience feelings of guilt or hopelessness. Sometimes people are so depressed they attempt suicide.

It is believed that bipolar mood disorder is caused by a combination of factors, such as genetics, biochemistry (a chemical imbalance in the brain) and stress. The seasons also seem to have an impact, as mania is more common in spring and depression more common in early winter.

Sources: The website of The Black Dog Institute <www. blackdoginstitute.org.au> and *What is Bipolar mood disorder?*, a brochure published by the Mental Health Branch of the Department of Health and Ageing, Canberra.

Contents

Introduction

Jamie Beggs started writing this book in 1994. Unsure where he wanted to be in life, he had taken time off work to travel the world and experience some other places and cultures to broaden his mind and increase his appreciation of life. His life had been normal and happy up to that time. Born in Ipswich, Queensland, Australia, on 17 November 1968, he was the second of three boys to Mary and Richard and is the middle brother to Andrew and Cameron. Jamie was an avid sportsman throughout his younger years and excelled in soccer and cricket. He had a wide circle of friends and was popular with the girls. After living in Malaysia for a few years, Jamie finished high school in Perth, Western Australia, in 1986. He worked a number of part-time jobs, before finding full-time employment at the R&I Bank as a teller. Jamie's good customer service and interpersonal skills quickly saw him promoted to a training and quality assessments team. Jamie continued to work at the R&I Bank until he became disillusioned with the banking vocation, resulting in him deciding to travel the world.

But Jamie's travels and life did not turn out as planned. He experienced a number of life-changing events over the years that have had a profound impact on his life, his family, and his friends. Just when it seemed he was on track to be successful and live a 'normal' life, he would be knocked down again, and again.

Inner Journey is Jamie's account of his experiences after his life changed and his struggle to understand his path in life. This book is Jamie's way to tell his story and prove that it is possible to overcome the obstacles in life and rise above all challenges.

The book was almost finished when Jamie's life was turned upside down once more in January 2004. Unfortunately, the book had to be finished by his family. What you are about to read is typed up from Jamie's own written work, with very minor editing by others.

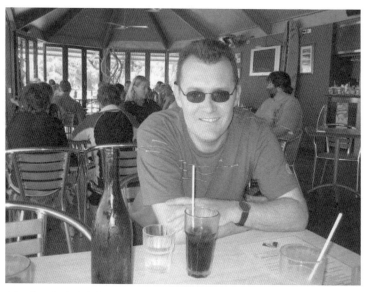

Me, Jamie (2006)

1

Spain

I was in Pamplona for San Fermin, a festival celebrated by the Spanish people for the patron saint of Pamplona and famous for the running of the bulls. I had been in Pamplona for some five days or so. I was actually on holidays from a teaching position I held in London. After five nights of enjoying the festivities I decided to have a relatively quiet night in comparison, as it was my intention to leave in the next few days and spend a few days lying on the beach in San Sebastian — a nearby town on the coast. I was with Neil, a work colleague who I had met up with some days prior, and we spent the night walking around the streets, taking in the atmosphere. The Spanish really did know how to have a good time as they danced in the street while brass bands were playing. After a week there weren't as many people as there had been earlier, when thousands of people had crammed the cobble-stoned streets, dressed in white with a red scarf, wearing the traditional colours of San Fermin. The bars had been overflowing with people, usually intoxicated after drinking the local sangria. Each day the tradition of running with the bulls had taken place, with hundreds of men running through the narrow streets, being chased by the bulls into the stadium. I had been the previous year with some other friends that I had travelled through Portugal and Spain with. I had experienced the rush of being chased by ten bulls through the streets, while people cheered or shook their heads, wondering why we would be crazy enough to do such a thing. They say that it is supposed to be a test of your manhood in Spanish culture to run with the bulls, so I'm not sure where that leaves me as I was definitely running *from* the bulls.

I had had such a good time the previous year that it didn't take too much convincing to come back again. I had already been away from Australia on a world trip for just over a year after travelling through America, the Cayman Islands, Canada and parts of southern Europe. I was having a great time away and was glad that I had achieved my dream of travelling the world. As I continued to walk around the streets with Neil we came across a couple of Spanish girls with whom we shared an apartment. We stopped and had a brief chat with them in Spanish, and organized to meet up with them later. The festival had given me the chance to use the Spanish I had studied while I was living in London. It was a great experience to be able to communicate with the Spanish people and gain an insight into their culture, even though my Spanish was admittedly limited.

As a result of speaking a lot of Spanish I was noticing that I was feeling quite tired mentally. I had also noticed over the time that I had spent at the festival that my thought processes had sped up from time to time. I remember as I was talking to Neil that I felt like getting away and that relaxing for a few days in San Sebastian would be a good idea. After talking to the girls, Neil and I decided we were going to head up to the mussel bar, which was a place where a number of Australians and New Zealanders met during the festival. As we were walking through the streets I recall feeling quite faint. I was having a general conversation with Neil about my trip and what I was planning on doing in the future. As I was talking, I once again noticed that my thought processes had begun to speed up. I explained to Neil that something was happening to me and that I would need to sit down. Neil said he would get me a glass of water from one of the bars along the street and I waited on a small fence on the side of the road. I continued to feel light-headed. Neil returned with a glass of water and I had a sip of the water and tried to get my thoughts together.

After five minutes or so I got off the fence and once again felt faint. The next thing that occurred was that my legs buckled under me and I collapsed, falling to the ground. I think I blacked out briefly, but found that upon regaining consciousness my thoughts were still racing. My thoughts were not unlike a tape recorder being sped up. By this time Neil had run off to call an ambulance. I remember finding it hard to gain control of my thoughts as I was beginning to panic, wondering what was happening to me. There were people gathered around where I had collapsed and I remember a Spanish girl speaking to me and holding my hand to comfort me. My body felt completely lifeless as I was lying on the side of the road, and by this point I felt I was going to die. I began praying that I wouldn't die and I felt as though I was fighting for my life — my thoughts were still racing and disordered. I couldn't move as my body felt like it was floating. I continued to pray in my mind, calling out for help and that I didn't want to die. It was after another minute or so that I felt volts of energy charge through my body and from lying on the ground feeling completely lifeless I was thrown into the air and onto my feet.

I was amazed to find myself back on my feet, but I noticed that my thoughts were still racing as I was trying to compose myself. I saw the ambulance that Neil had called and thought that it would be wise to go to the hospital. I got into the back of the ambulance when two paramedics yelled *"tranquilo"* ("calm down"); I must have shown them that I was startled by what had just happened. I rode in the back of the ambulance, still trying to gain control of my thoughts. I found that my thoughts had become disconnected and I had the perception of hearing voices. I was becoming restless as I found myself experiencing what was later described to me as a psychotic episode.

I became very paranoid as I arrived at the hospital and my thinking had become disordered. I was now actually quite frightened by what I had just been through. Neil had been in the front of the ambulance and was walking into the hospital with me when my paranoia increased and I felt I had to get away from the hospital. I was overwhelmed with fear as I ran through the streets, still hearing voices and finding it difficult to gain control of my thoughts. I ran, not knowing where I was going, just barely managing to avoid the oncoming traffic. Neil ran after me, noticing that I was scared, and when I eventually stopped he approached me with caution, allowing me time to calm down. I was breathing heavily after running for over a kilometre to get away from the hospital. Neil continued to talk to me, telling me to remain calm. I was starting to gain more control after what felt like wrestling for power over my thoughts. I was beginning to breathe more evenly but now felt dehydrated and gestured to Neil that I needed some water. We found a café not far from where I had stopped running and by this time I sat down quite calmly and drank some water. I was frightened by the whole experience, trying to understand what had just happened. Neil, who obviously found it difficult to comprehend my behaviour, continued to reassure me that everything was all right.

I no longer had the perception of hearing voices as I continued to drink water. After ten minutes or so we decided it would probably be best to make our way back to the flat where we were staying in Pamplona. Neil actually felt I should go back to the hospital but I thought getting back to the flat and lying down would help and felt that I was more in control. Because I had run away from the hospital we found ourselves in a district that was unfamiliar. We continued walking until we came into familiar territory. When we eventually arrived back at the flat I sat down in the kitchen, still in a state of shock. I continued to drink water in an effort to rehydrate myself. I explained to Neil how confused I was by the experience. He suggested it would probably be best if we got some sleep, and we decided to go to bed.

I found I was unable to sleep, trying to make some sense of everything that had happened. I was lying on the bed and my thoughts were concentrated on how it was possible that I was flung into the air after being pinned to the ground. I was convinced that I had had some kind of near-death experience and felt frustrated that I didn't seem to have the answers. I looked over towards the window and noticed that it was becoming lighter outside as the sun began to rise. I could still hear the brass bands playing in the streets as the Spaniards continued to party. Neil and I shared the same room and Neil seemed to be reflecting on everything I had said earlier and also wasn't able to sleep. I told Neil how I felt I had come close to dying and was feeling relieved that I was still alive. I told him that I was going to contact my Spanish girlfriend, Eva, whom I had met in London while teaching English to foreign students there. Eva had stayed in London to continue her study and her part-time job as sales assistant in a shoe store.

I called Eva early that morning to catch her before she went off to work. After being connected through by the operator, I heard the phone begin to ring and then I heard Eva's voice. It was good to hear a familiar, friendly voice. She seemed a bit surprised at the call and could probably detect that I was somewhat distant. I decided not to mention what had happened during the night as I was still unsure of how to explain what had occurred and I didn't want to upset her. I simply said I was missing her and looking forward to seeing her when I returned to London. After saying goodbye to Eva I made my way back to the bedroom and lay back down on the bed.

I found I was still unable to sleep, as I was thinking about the nightmare I had just experienced. I was becoming anxious once again and my thoughts were starting to race. After another hour or so I began thinking that I would need to talk to a doctor and I asked Neil if he could call the hospital to arrange for an ambulance to be sent. I waited in the bedroom and could hear Neil talking in Spanish to the hospital. I was only able to understand the basics of what he was saying as my level of Spanish was below intermediate. Whilst Neil was talking on the phone I heard the doorbell ring. The apartment we were staying in had about six bedrooms, all of which were empty except for the room we were in and one other room occupied by two young Spanish girls. One of the girls went to answer the door whilst Neil continued to talk on the telephone. I heard an older Spanish couple talking as they entered the apartment. Although I wasn't able to fully understand what was being said, it was clear by the tone of their voices that they weren't happy. I asked Neil if he could explain what was going on. As it turned out, they were the owners of the apartment and they were angry that they hadn't been told about me staying in the students' apartments. I walked into the kitchen where they were standing and tried to explain how I was a friend of one of the students and thought that they had been notified. I apologized for the misunderstanding with the help of Neil and said we would vacate the apartment.

Meanwhile, one of the girls told me the ambulance had arrived. I made my way down the stairs with Neil and was met by the paramedics. I was quite agitated by everything that had happened and felt getting to the hospital would give me a chance to talk to a psychiatrist and hopefully get some answers. As we arrived at the hospital I felt more composed than I had been the night before and I waited as Neil went to register me as a patient. It wasn't too long before I heard my name called by a doctor wearing a white overcoat, and along with Neil I followed him into a room. We sat down in a small room with a couple of chairs and a bed. I asked if the doctor could speak any English, which he unfortunately was unable to do. I used my basic Spanish and the help of Neil to try and explain what had happened to me over the course of the night. It was very difficult to explain to the doctor what I had experienced, as I was admittedly quite confused by what had happened. I mentioned how I had experienced racing thoughts as well as having the perception of hearing voices. The doctor appeared to be equally confused by what I was saying. He felt that I would need to stay in hospital for a period of time so that I could be given some treatment. He noticed that I was fairly agitated by the experience and thought a sedative would help me get some sleep.

I was placed on a hospital bed to be wheeled up to the ward. I felt very tired as a result of the sedative and the lack of sleep, and I began to dose off. I slept for a few hours before being woken up by a pain in my back. It was one of the doctors doing a lumbar puncture to test my cerebrospinal fluid. I dosed off again and next woke up in a hospital room that had been darkened by the curtains being closed. I was confused for a moment, wondering where I was and still finding it difficult to gain control of my thoughts. I then saw the door being opened and a female doctor walked into the room, speaking in Spanish. I wasn't able to understand what she was saying to me. She then said in English "voices, are you hearing voices?" I felt so drowsy and still wasn't able to gain total control of my thoughts, but nodded my head in acknowledgement. I told the doctor in Spanish that I had a severe headache and tried to explain that I felt nauseous. I hadn't eaten anything for quite some time and I wasn't sure if I would be able to hold anything down. After another five minutes or so a nurse came into the room with some aspirin to help with my headache. I then tried to get to sleep again, as I felt almost haunted by the memories of what had happened the night before.

I was later woken up by the curtains being pulled. The nurse said I had a visitor. It was Neil, who asked how I was feeling. It was good to hear someone speaking in English. I asked him where I was and he explained that I was in the psychiatric ward of the hospital. I felt ashamed and embarrassed to be there. I seemed to have more control of my thoughts by this stage, but I was still feeling quite nauseous. It felt like there was a lot of pressure on my head, particularly behind my eyes, and my head continued to pound. Neil explained that he was going to have to head back to London soon to return to work. He told me that he had been in contact with Eva in London and had explained what had happened. He said that she was quite upset and was going to come down to the hospital in Pamplona to be with me for a while.

After speaking to Neil for some time I felt it was time I got into contact with my mum and dad in Australia, to let them know what had happened. I really didn't know what I was going to say to my mum, who, like most mothers, wouldn't like to hear that her son was in the psychiatric ward of a Spanish hospital. I asked one of the nurses if I could use a telephone and then Neil helped with the connection. I heard the phone ring and then my mother's voice. I tried to explain as calmly as I could the predicament I was in. I was still finding it difficult to get control of my thoughts. Mum and dad were understandably upset and I can remember mum saying that she had felt something was wrong. Mum is always able to sense when something is wrong, whether it be with me or either of my two brothers. The conversation didn't last very long and I wasn't able to communicate as effectively as I would have liked, which I now know only made them worry all the more. After hanging up and speaking to my mum, dad and younger brother, I was led back to my room with the understanding that they had the essential information that I was unwell, that I was in a hospital in Pamplona in Spain, and that I would be in contact with them again soon.

While leading me back to my room one of the psychiatric

nurses was talking to me in Spanish. The fact that I didn't have a clue what she was saying didn't seem to matter. As she continued, I noticed the surroundings of the ward. It was quite frightening to see the people in the ward dealing with their own psychiatric problems. I can remember one woman in a wheelchair sitting in the corridor with her arm raised in the air screaming, and other people walking up and down the corridor. I was glad that I had a private room. I was feeling very lethargic as I walked back to my room and I was getting frustrated by the language barrier and finding it difficult to communicate with the nurses. I was starting to wonder what was wrong with me as my head felt like it was ready to explode with the pressure that had built up. I lay back down on the bed and tried to get more sleep. I was still quite sedated and as a result felt myself drowsing from time to time. I would occasionally eat the food that was being brought in but found myself vomiting up most of what I ate. I was losing all of my energy, and making my way to the toilet was becoming more and more difficult.

I was looking forward to Eva arriving to help overcome the language barrier. I could tell that the nurses were also becoming frustrated, as the majority were unable to speak any English. I can still remember one particular incident when I went to have a shower and because of my lack of energy I sat on the floor in the shower. I had tried to ask for a chair in Spanish but the nurse obviously couldn't understand me, and after fifteen minutes or so she returned to find me still sitting on the floor, while the shower flooded the bathroom with water pouring out onto the carpet. The nurse yelled abuse at me, which I was fortunately unable to understand, as I'm sure it wasn't kind. It wasn't long after that that I got my chair.

2

Family

After what would have been a week or so that I had been in hospital I awoke one morning to the bright smiling face of Eva, who had just arrived from London. Eva had distinctly Spanish features and a permanent smile. She was very concerned to find I was in hospital and asked me what had happened. I once again tried to explain what had occurred over the previous few days and that I was feeling very tired as a result of what I had been through. Having Eva at the hospital made it so much easier to communicate with the nurses and doctors. Eva spoke to some of the doctors who had been treating me and advised me that I had only been given sedatives to that point to enable me to sleep. The doctors weren't sure of a diagnosis and as a result didn't want to prescribe anything stronger.

I was feeling a lot better mentally and felt I was in control of my thoughts. I was still finding it difficult to keep anything down and the doctors were still unsure as to why that was. I found I was sleeping a lot of the time and would generally wake up around meal times. Because I was continually vomiting, a different doctor came in to examine me and try to ascertain exactly what was wrong with me. I remember being taken to a different part of the hospital in a wheelchair for further examinations. The doctor who was examining me spoke English, which made things easier. It was quite funny to hear him talk, as he was a Spanish doctor but actually spoke English with an Irish accent. He explained that from the tests that had been done they still weren't able to determine why I was continually vomiting. He said that he felt there was a neurological problem that had to be investigated and that a neurologist was going to be coming to see me.

I had been in hospital for almost two weeks by this stage and I was still in the psychiatric ward. The neurologist eventually came to see me, along with a number of young trainee doctors. He was explaining to the students the background of my case and the treatment I had been given and the students as well as the doctor seemed to be perplexed. I had been told by the doctor through Eva as an interpreter that the cranial pressure I was experiencing was usually due to a thrombosis. The doctor explained that there was evidence of a papilledema, which is a swelling of the optic disk. He was unsure of a definite diagnosis as a series of brain scans hadn't shown any evidence of a thrombosis. The doctor said that I would need to be transferred to the neurological ward where I could be given further treatment.

After two weeks Eva said that she was going to have to return to London to work. She said that she had been in contact with another friend of mine in London, Steve, who was going to come down to be with me for a week.

Meanwhile, my family had been calling from Australia to try and get an update on my condition. I was unaware of the problems they were experiencing with the language barrier and they weren't able to get any conclusive answers on my condition. It was only later that I found out that they were beside themselves with worry and that they were planning on coming over to Spain.

Eva had been great in the time she had spent looking after me. It had certainly made it easier to communicate with the doctors.

Eva was quite emotional as she left to return to England. I think being at the hospital had proved to be pretty draining for her. She said she would be in contact when she arrived in London.

I was fortunate that I had a few friends in London and not long after Eva left Steve arrived. I had first met Steve while travelling in the Greek Islands; we got talking and immediately hit it off. He was one of the nicest guys I had met in a long time.

Steve came down to the hospital in the third week and by this stage I was feeling very weak and had lost a lot of weight. I had managed to find out from a nurse in the neurological ward that the doctors were still unsure of a diagnosis, as the tests that had been done hadn't shed any light on the problem. Steve had continued to care for me, helping me into the shower and giving me words of encouragement. Eventually the doctor placed me on an intravenous drip. I had been moved to the neurological ward and was sharing the room with an older Spanish man. I was beginning to feel better as a result of being on the drip and I talked with the man's wife who was by his side through the night and also looking after me. I was lucky to have so many people caring for me. I was quite frightened, not knowing what was wrong with me, and it had crossed my mind a number of times that I was fortunate to still be alive.

After the fourth week I was told that that my mum and brother would be arriving soon. It was only later that I found out that mum had experienced problems getting a visa to be able to enter Spain. When they eventually arrived they were very tired from the long flight and worried about the state they would find me in. I felt terrible about them having to make the trip to Spain and all the worry that I had caused. My dad and other brother and my extended family were also worried to hear that I had been in hospital in Spain for four weeks.

Mum and Cameron came just as Steve was leaving after looking after me for a week. It was good to see them despite the circumstances, as I hadn't seen them for quite some time. We talked about what we should do and we decided that because of the language problems in Spain it would be wise to go to England and continue the treatment there.

Meanwhile, over the few days that mum and Cameron came to visit me at the hospital, mum, despite the language barrier, developed a friendship with the Spanish lady who was caring for her husband. Mum would always give the lady a hug and comfort her and thank her for being there and also looking after me.

When the doctor came to give me a final check-up for discharge, I was still feeling lethargic and sick. I had stopped vomiting but had noticed that when I opened my bowels there was some blood. I knew I wasn't well enough to be discharged but we all felt that it would be better to get to England. Eventually, the doctor reluctantly signed a discharge letter detailing the treatment that I had been given.

I found it hard to walk because of my lack of energy, so a nurse wheeled me out of the hospital in a wheelchair to a waiting taxi. We went back to where my mum and Cameron were staying and we knew that we would all have to make our way up to Bilbao in the north of Spain in the Basque country so that we could catch a plane to London. We caught a bus to the Bilbao airport, with mum and Cam supporting me along the way. After finding someone that could speak English I got a wheelchair and we made our way through customs and onto the plane. It was a relief to be finally leaving Spain after what had turned out to be a nightmare.

I was beginning to reflect on everything that had happened over the past few weeks and trying to understand it. I was thinking back to when it all began during the festival and how it had turned my life upside down. The whole experience was already making me think differently. I was starting to question what had happened. I was convinced I'd had some kind of near-death experience.

I tried to explain to my mum what had happened and how lucky I felt I had been. Mum and I share a very close bond and she felt it may have happened for a reason and that my life had possibly been heading down the wrong road. Mum feels things all happen for a reason and that we are all on our own paths for a purpose. I felt as though I had been given a jolt to make me stop and think as to where my life was heading and what the purpose of my life was.

I wouldn't have considered myself to be a spiritual person up to that point in my life. I never really asked deeper, more meaningful questions about our existence, but after what had occurred I experienced a kind of spiritual awakening. I felt a presence that I can't quite explain as I lay on the side of road in Spain. I felt as though I was helped, and since I am more spiritually aware. Before I always thought more scientifically but after what I experienced feel that there is a spiritual realm. As I sat on the plane and we made our way to England, with me still unsure of what was wrong with me, I tried to remain in a positive mindset and had faith that whatever it was, it would be discovered.

We arrived in London after a one-hour flight. The first thing we did was to organise to go to a hospital in Hampstead. It was immediately noticeable that things were made easier without the Spanish language as an obstacle. The doctor was given the discharge letter that had been written by the neurologist in Spain. He appeared to be able to understand most of what was written. I remember he was quite a young doctor. He examined me in the emergency area, checking for the papilledema that he had just read about. After some 20 minutes or so I heard him say that I would have to be referred to a specialist. I can remember the look on my mum's face, knowing that there was nothing that the doctor could do, and that it would be difficult getting to see a specialist.

I was still very tired and weak and I was to later realise it was quite surprising that the doctor actually allowed me to leave the hospital under mum's care. He said that a letter detailing when an appointment could be set up with the specialist would be sent to Eva's address. That letter arrived after a couple of days, stating that the earliest appointment possible, due to the pressures on the English health system, would not be for another three months. We were all concerned and realised that the only thing to do was to try to get a flight back to Australia. The obvious next concern was whether my condition would worsen over a long flight. We spoke to a few doctors, asking whether flying would have an adverse effect. Their responses were non-committal and they were not prepared to sign off on anything. Mum and Cam discussed the situation with me and we all decided that we would have to take the chance. There was no way that we could wait (or afford to wait) three months. Cam made the preparations to fly back to Australia as soon as possible.

At this time, I realised that my travels had come to an end. Mum always said that things happen for a reason.

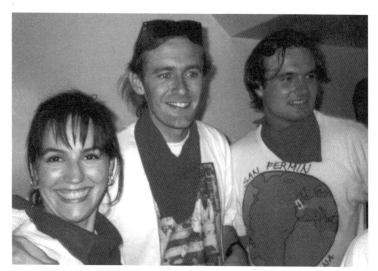

Me with Neil and a Spanish friend, celebrating San Fermin, Pamplona, Spain

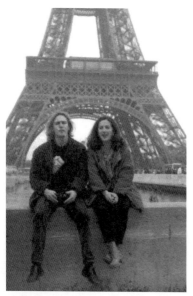

With Eva in Paris

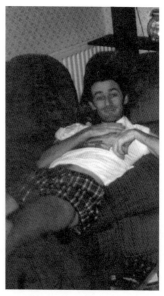

Just out of hospital…

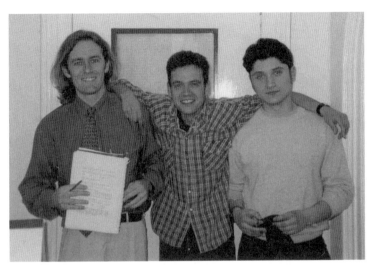

Me (left) with two of my students at Callan College, London

3

Australia

It felt so good to touch down in Australia. The flight back to Australia had lasted over 20 hours. I was weak and tired but got through the flight without any further complications. Cam had managed to convince the hostesses to give me an area of three seats so that I could get some rest. Needless to say, I ate little and drank only water.

I was concerned about mum and Cam but I was looking forward to seeing my dad. I knew he had been quite worried, and that he had his own health problems to contend with. I had spoken to him a few times over the course of the month but it must have been difficult for him to get an accurate picture of exactly what had happened. He was waiting at the airport and I could see the relief on his face when we made our way out of the arrivals gate. My dad had experienced bad health just after he retired from the Royal Australian Air Force. He had kidney failure and heart complications, which nearly took him from us. He became very ill and waited a few years for a transplant. He never really recovered physically, losing a lot of weight and strength. He was essentially half the man he used to be, and the last thing he needed was to be worried about me.

Upon our arrival in Australia, the plan was to make me an appointment with a neurologist as soon as possible. Mum had been making all the calls and within a couple of days, I was booked in. I recall getting a thorough examination at which time the neurologist also detected the papilledema. He was shocked that I had travelled in my condition and that I hadn't been treated sooner. He explained in clinical terms how the papilledema was due to an increase in cranial pressure and that I would need immediate treatment. This was the second time that I realised that I was lucky to be alive. I was promptly transferred to a hospital in Perth for further tests and probable surgery. There was an immediate need to relieve the pressure in my head. They conducted a lumbar puncture in the lower part of my spine. I later learned that this was to reduce the intracranial pressure caused by an excess of cerebrospinal fluid on the brain.

The neurologist ordered that a series of MRIs be conducted to determine the cause or origin of the problem. Results over the next few days revealed that I had sagittal sinus thrombosis. Apparently the technology and equipment used back in the Spanish hospital was not capable of detecting this condition.

The neurologist explained that I would have to have a series of lumbar punctures to ensure the intracranial pressure was maintained at a normal level. The lumbar punctures were extremely painful. The doctor would insert a large needle into the lumbar sack at the base of the spine and draw out fluid. This was done while I was lying on my side in the foetal position, which I had to do two to three times a week. This was necessary while they waited for the thrombosis to dissipate. I had no alternative but to put up with the pain of those excruciating needles.

It was two weeks before they would discharge me from the hospital. I continued treatment as an outpatient, coming in to the hospital about three times a week. I was feeling better as a result of the lumbar punctures, but the fact that I continued having them week after week, meant that the thrombosis still hadn't dissipated. A little while later I was told I had another problem, which was occurring because of the pressure on my brain. It had caused the optic disc to swell resulting in pressure on the optic nerve. I had noticed that my peripheral vision was being affected but I put this down to normal migraine symptoms. This added to my anxiety, knowing that without treating the thrombosis I could go blind.

In the time that I was being treated as an outpatient, I was living with my parents. The fact that I had lost a lot of weight and didn't have any energy meant that I spent most of my days at home, lying down watching videos. I would occasionally get some exercise by walking around the block, but I was quite often too exhausted. This routine, and returning to the hospital for those lumbar punctures and waiting for the thrombosis to dissipate, continued for months.

Eva had remained in England and I received letters from her each week. She was planning on coming down to Australia when she was able to obtain a working visa. I was thankful to have Eva to support me. She really was a tower of strength. I was also lucky to have good friends in Perth that I had grown up with who offered their support.

The time that I spent as an outpatient gave me an opportunity to try to reflect on what had happened. I kept returning to the time I was in the psychiatric ward of the hospital and my perception of hearing voices. My mental health whilst I was being treated as an outpatient seemed to be good. It was as if the disturbance of thought that I had experienced had been so traumatic that it had gone into my subconscious. I was able to think quite clearly during this period of time. I was still feeling worried as I continued to have treatment for the thrombosis. I was finding it difficult to sleep at night and I could feel the increased cranial pressure. I was also more aware that my vision was affected as a result of the pressure on the optic nerve.

It was during this time that I really began to do some soul-searching. Up until this point in my life I had lived a fairly normal life. I hadn't really encountered any major problems. I had a loving, supportive family as well as a number of good friends. I had always enjoyed life and never really been challenged up to that point. Now I felt as though I was about to climb a mountain, and I hadn't had any prior climbing experience.

The first step was to hope that the thrombosis would dissipate as this would diminish the anxiety I was experiencing. As the days went by I continued having the lumbar punctures and my spare time was spent reading. I was taking medication to reduce the amount of cerebrospinal fluid being produced by my brain. Even with the medication my intracranial pressure continued to be high, which necessitated more lumbar punctures. After a number of months of receiving treatment as an outpatient the neurologist told me that there was an alternative to continually having lumbar punctures. He explained that there was an operation that could be done which would involve a peritoneal shunt being inserted into the lumbar sack. This shunt would act as a pressure valve, draining excess cerebrospinal fluid into the peritoneal cavity. The neurologist explained that this was only usually used as a last resort if the thrombosis hadn't dissipated.

Eventually, after some four months had passed and over thirty lumbar punctures had been done, the decision was made to go ahead and operate. An appointment was made to see a neurosurgeon. It was quite frightening at the time but it appeared to be the only option rather than continually having lumbar punctures. The neurosurgeon examined me and said that I would be operated on as soon as possible as it was a serious condition. I was readmitted to hospital within the next few days. The operation itself was quite complex and scheduled to take between two and three hours.

The night before the operation I was feeling quite anxious at the prospect of having such a major operation. I was finding it difficult to sleep and eventually asked the nurse for something to help me do so. When I awoke early the next morning my parents were in the room, waiting to keep me company before the operation. It was about 6.00am when the orderly came into my room to wheel me down to the operating theatre. It wasn't too long before I was saying goodbye to my mum and dad and taken to see the anaesthetist. The next thing I remember was being asked to count to ten and only making it to about four.

After what seemed like no more than a few minutes I became conscious and I found myself in Recovery. There was a nurse by my bedside who was giving me injections of morphine to kill the pain. Even with the morphine the pain was excruciating. It wasn't too long before my mum and dad came into the recovery area, providing words of encouragement and saying that it was all over. I was amazed at how quickly everything seemed to have happened. I was still feeling very groggy and my thoughts were concentrated on the pain I was feeling. After a little while I was taken back up to my room. Mum and dad were still with me and being very supportive.

I was told by the neurologist that I would be kept in hospital for some time until I had recovered from the operation. He said that everything had gone well. I was relieved that it was over but I noticed that I was still feeling the anxiety I had experienced prior to the operation. I started to notice that, just as I had felt in Spain some four months previously, I was beginning to lose control of my thoughts once again. The perception in my mind of hearing voices returned. I was in the neurology ward of the hospital and as well as hearing voices I became so anxious that I was finding it difficult to breath and had to be placed on a respirator. The nurses and doctors were unsure of what was happening.

I remember my mum and dad talking to me, saying that I had to try and take control of myself. I was finding it more and more difficult as my thoughts became disordered. It had become noticeable that I was incoherent and that, as I first thought, the trauma I had suffered in Spain had in fact gone into my subconscious. The operation and possibly the morphine that I had been given appeared to cause the nightmare I had experienced in Spain to come flooding back into my consciousness. I was paranoid, delusional and once again thought I heard voices. It really felt as though I had gotten lost in my mind for a period of time. I was constantly losing control of my thoughts. I remember being transferred to the psychiatric ward of the hospital and talking to a psychiatrist. I can only vaguely remember some of the conversations I had with the doctors as they tried to make a diagnosis. I was feeling very paranoid and remember thinking that everyone was against me and out to harm me.

I had been in the psychiatric ward of the hospital for a week or so before I was eventually transferred to a mental hospital as an involuntary patient. It was at this time that I did the deepest of my soul-searching. I really felt as though I was lost, and that mountain I was climbing was even bigger than I thought. I was now having to deal with something that I felt at that time was well beyond me. I can remember my parents coming in to visit me from time to time and occasionally answering the phone calls from friends who were concerned. I only have a vague recollection of a lot of what happened during my first week in hospital. As I later found out, the doctors were treating me for symptoms of schizophrenia as it was common to have the perception of hearing voices with this particular illness. I was heavily sedated, which made it very difficult for me to communicate with anyone. I remember that at this time I felt as though I had really gone into myself. It was almost as if I was regressing to my childhood, becoming withdrawn as a result of everything that had happened to me. It was like I was trying to find the real me and I was finding that as a I hadn't been challenged with any adversity to that point in my life I didn't have a lot strength to draw on. I found I was really leaning on my parents during this time.

Mum and dad were coming to the hospital every day and spending hours supporting me as I was confronted with one obstacle after another. It's only now that I look back on that time that I realise how much I drew on my parent's strength as they were supporting me through the hardest time of my life. As a result I've found that I share an even closer bond with them.

I once read that being spiritual and accepting peace in your mind allowed you to get closer to your soul. I felt at this time I was the closest I had been to my soul and it was during this dark time that I felt as though I was being guided. Whilst I was in hospital my aunt Pam bought me a book of metaphysical quotations. I used this book to help me through these hard times. A quote from Carl Jung was one particular quote that helped:

> "Even a happy life cannot be without a measure of darkness and the word 'happiness' would lose its meaning if it were not balanced by sadness".
>
> *Carl Jung*

I began to view this experience as a journey of self-discovery.

I had been in hospital for a month. The doctors were reluctant to make a definite diagnosis and, as I later realised, it was difficult for doctors given the fact that I was so confused by everything that had happened. As I had been delusional, paranoid and had the perception of hearing voices, a form of schizophrenia was the label given to my condition. I felt frightened at possibly being a schizophrenic as I admittedly shared in the misinformed view that schizophrenics were dangerous. I wasn't able to accept that I had schizophrenia and my feelings were influenced by the stigma that existed.

Whatever it was that was wrong with me, I was in a state of denial. I continued somewhat reluctantly to take the medication that had been prescribed and after what had been almost two months of being hospitalised I felt more in control. I was able to communicate with my parents who had continued to visit me everyday. I still felt sedated the whole time I was in the mental hospital and I kept pretty much to myself. I would occasionally talk to some of the other patients but found that the majority of them due to their own illnesses didn't want to be befriended. Graylands hospital was the largest public mental hospital in Perth and consisted of a number of different wards. There were locked wards where involuntary patients like myself received treatment. The wards were given names and the particular ward that you were admitted to appeared to be dependent upon the severity of your illness. I found myself in three different wards during my time in hospital. When my illness was at its worst I was in the acute care ward where there were less patients and this meant the nurses were able to spend more time caring for the patients. I once heard the hospital described as "the palace" by one of the patients, when in actual fact it was a dreary, orange-bricked, depressing structure that felt more like a prison. Graylands had a terrible reputation for housing the worst of the mentally ill in Perth, and I knew I had to get out of there as soon as I could.

When the doctor felt I had improved I was eventually transferred to the open ward. You were allowed to come and go as you pleased in the open ward and there was only limited supervision. I took the opportunity to get out of there whenever I could and it gave me the opportunity to spend the days at home with mum and dad rather than staying at the hospital. I would return to the hospital at night despite my protests to my family that I didn't want to go back. I can remember one occasion when my brother Andrew drove me back to the hospital. Andrew is a couple of years older than I and is a security policeman in the air force. He had recently been posted back to Perth and it was good to have his support. On this particular occasion the time I had spent in hospital had really taken its toll and I said to Andrew I didn't want to go back in there. I was crying as I said it and he gave me a firm hug and assured me that it would be all over soon. It felt like my life had become a nightmare that I was unable to awaken from. I found my family to be supportive although no one seemed to fully understand the pain I was going through. I appeared to be suffering from post-traumatic stress as a result of the psychotic episode I had first experienced in Spain as well as reliving the psychoses that I had experienced as a result of the operation. I felt like I only had myself and continued to have faith that I would eventually escape from the darkness and see the light.

But one morning it all got too much to take. I vaguely remember getting up and making my way to the bathroom. The stress on me and my family must have made me lose control and just want to end this nightmare. I looked around and found my disposable razor. I just thought that I could cut my wrists and it would all be over. I recall pushing and sliding the blade on my wrists in the hope that I could get deep enough to cut the veins. It wasn't working. I could see the blood on both wrists but the blade couldn't cut deep enough. I cried and groaned with frustration. That's when my father walked in to the bathroom, calling my name. He must have seen the cubicle door slightly open and pushed it further and saw me lying on the ground. He screamed out my name and then reached over and pushed the emergency button. I remember parts of what happened after that, where dad was yelling for help, putting some towels on my wrists, while still trying to give me words of encouragement. The nurses had rushed in and soon taken over from dad to check on the extent of bleeding. They then took me back to my room to finish tending to the cuts and giving me a sedative. The rest of the day was spent with people and nurses checking up on me before I was moved to the acute care ward. This is where all the suicidal patients or untrustworthy ones were sent until they could prove they were no longer a danger to themselves or others. I was in this ward for a few weeks, and it made me realise how bad things really were.

There were times during this period that I felt like giving up but something kept me going. My family would visit regularly with words of support and little gifts of food and drink. My family really were my pillar of strength. And they never again commented on my attempted suicide.

I also kept receiving letters of encouragement from Eva who was still planning on coming to Australia to be with me. I was beginning to think that it would be too much for Eva to take on and remember asking mum to write her a letter telling her not to come. Mum understood how I felt, yet Eva insisted that she still wanted to come to Australia and said how much she was missing me.

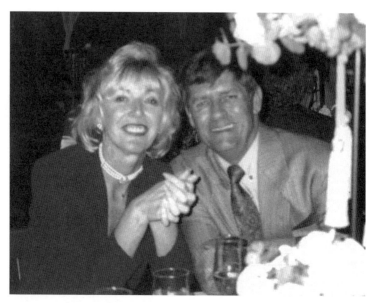

Mum and Dad, Perth, Western Australia, 2001

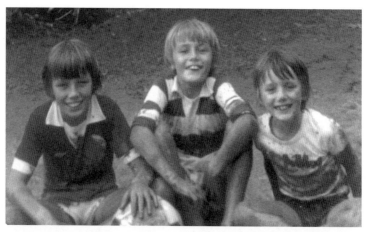

From left to right, Andrew, me and Cameron, Penang,
Malaysia, 1978

4

Eva arrives...

Towards the end of my stay in the hospital, Eva finally arrived in Perth. It had been some six months since I had seen her and I tried to put on a front that I wasn't as unwell as I actually was. Eva wasn't worried by the fact that I was in a mental hospital and said how happy she was to see me. She was like a breath of fresh air and her love gave me the boost that I was needing after months of depression. It wasn't too long after Eva arrived that I was discharged from hospital.

Eva was staying with mum and dad and until she was able to find work we both stayed there. I was given some medication upon my release. It felt like I had just come out of prison and I made a promise to myself that I would never go back. My mind was still feeling very fragile as a result of everything I had been through. I viewed it as though I had a broken leg and I still had a caste on and it would take time to heal completely. The thing was that I was unsure of exactly what lay ahead for my recovery and whether my mind would feel normal again. It was difficult to know exactly what normal was, as my life had been turned upside down and I couldn't really remember how I felt prior to the breakdown.

Eva and I felt it would be good to move out of mum and dad's place so I could then try and regain some independence. The first few weeks that I spent with Eva were wonderful. Although we hadn't known each other for a particularly long period of time I felt very comfortable with her. We were both very happy and enjoyed each other's company, taking walks along the beach and spending nights together having quiet dinners or relaxing watching videos. Eva was always in a happy mood and loved everything about life. She had an outgoing personality and despite the fact that English was her second language she made every effort to get to know my family and friends. She was a very strong person which made it easier for me during my recovery as she was very supportive. It didn't take too long before we found a house to share close to the city. Eva found work in a Spanish restaurant as a waitress. She really enjoyed the work and it gave her the opportunity to meet other Spanish people in Perth. Because of her friendly nature it didn't take long for her to build up a network of friends.

I found myself in a difficult position with what I was going to do for work. Prior to my world trip I had been working in a bank for six years. As I thought about my future I tried to remain in a positive mindset. I could feel that I wasn't able to do any work that was going to be particularly stressful. During the first month of living with Eva in Australia I found I was still suffering from a bit of shock at the whole ordeal. It's only now that I realise that at that particular point in time I was still very confused by what had happened. I wasn't sure what to make of the diagnosis that had been given by the psychiatrist. I hadn't had the perception of hearing voices as I continued to take the medication prescribed.

I found that as a result of everything that had happened I was hungry to learn more about the mind and how it actually works. I wanted to gain more of an understanding and hopefully come up with some answers. I decided to study some psychology, which I found helpful. However, I discovered that psychology is based on a number of theories, so it was therefore difficult to know the truth as the mind and the inner workings of the brain in some respects remain a mystery. Looking back on that period I remember really being in denial about having any sort of illness. I thought that what I had experienced was a brief psychotic episode and at that time felt I had seen the last of the nightmare. I continued to study psychology by correspondence in an effort to gain more of an insight into what had happened. I felt at that early stage as though I was working on a giant jigsaw puzzle, trying to put all of the pieces together. I found it difficult to study as my concentration was affected and as a result it was difficult to read for long periods of time.

I talked about everything that had happened to me with Eva and explained how I was still confused by certain aspects of the experience. There was a park across the road from where we were living and Eva and I would quite often take walks at night and talk. We both shared a similar view when it came to spirituality in that we felt there was something but didn't feel there was need to practise a particular religion. I tried to explain my near-death experience and the profound effect it had had on me. I found talking to Eva helped although the language barrier did at times prove difficult. When we talked on a deeper level it was sometimes difficult for her to grasp everything. This made me determined that I would learn Spanish and between our English and Spanish we would be able to bridge the gap that existed.

I found as time went by the differences in our cultures made it difficult for the relationship to develop to a higher level. I sensed that Eva was frustrated, just as I was, yet we still cared for each other. Eva had been in Australia for some six months and she said how she was missing her family and friends in Spain. We spoke about the future and in particular how she was going to have to leave Australia at the expiry of her working visa. I still had very strong feelings for Eva and I was having to think seriously about the future and what I was going to do. My mental health had improved and I had been seeing a psychiatrist on a regular basis.

I talked to the psychiatrist about the experience In Spain and whether there was a possibility of a relapse. He was under the impression that it was a brief psychotic episode, possibly brought on by stress, and he felt I could have the medication phased out and over a period of time. This came as a relief in some ways as I felt it gave me more freedom to make plans for the future. The psychiatrist didn't feel I displayed the normal symptoms of schizophrenia and was therefore advised that provided I could look after my general health I shouldn't have any problems.

In the year that Eva spent in Australia she continued to work as a waitress as well as give private Spanish lessons. I continued to study Spanish and psychology and decided that upon the expiry of Eva's visa I would go back to Spain so that the relationship could continue. I thought that living in Spain would give me the opportunity to improve my Spanish and also enable me to get some work teaching English.

Eventually the decision was made that I would spend a year in Spain with Eva before deciding any further on our future. I was twenty-seven by this stage and happy that I felt I had made the right decision. The intention was for Eva to go over to Spain and find some work and get herself set up prior to me meeting up with her. Before Eva left we had a going away party at the house which gave everyone the opportunity to say goodbye to her. The number of people that Eva had met in the year she spent in Australia was amazing. She became quite emotional not knowing whether she would see a lot of her friends again.

Before too long the day that she was due to leave arrived. I took her to the airport with some friends and we bade her farewell. She was once again quite upset but knew that I would come over to Spain in the not too distant future.

Eva left for Spain just prior to Christmas and I moved out of the house we were sharing, back in with mum and dad until it was time for me to make my way to Spain. Soon I had a phone call from Eva saying she had arrived in Spain. I could hear the excitement in her voice, being happy to be back with her family and friends. She said that she didn't feel it would take too long before she would find some work. I was feeling excited yet also somewhat apprehensive at returning to Spain after my last experience. I was feeling healthy mentally and therefore didn't foresee that I would encounter any of the same problems again.

It had been about a month since I'd seen Eva, during which time I had enjoyed spending Christmas with my family and friends. I continued to get phone calls from Eva and she said that she had found some work in Valencia in the east of Spain. Knowing that Eva had found work, I went to book my ticket and planned to leave within a few weeks.

I was at home one night during the week just before I was due to leave for Spain when the phone rang. Mum answered and said it was from Spain but that it wasn't Eva. I was a little confused at who it would be as I answered the call. On the other end of the line I heard a Spanish girl struggling to speak English saying that she had some bad news. I didn't know what she was talking about when she said that Eva had been in a car accident and the next thing she said was that she had died. I was numb with shock after hearing this and my mum noticed immediately that there was something wrong. I dropped the phone from my grasp, repeating to my mum and dad that Eva had been killed in a car accident. Mum took the receiver and spoke to the girl, thinking it was some kind of cruel joke. But slowly it sank in that it was the horrible truth, Eva had died.

5

Melbourne

The only time in my life that I had someone close to me die was when my grandfather passed away. He had died whilst I was in England and it was a shock, but nothing compared to the numbing feeling after hearing that Eva had been killed in a car accident. It just didn't seem real. I couldn't believe how she had had her life taken from her at the age of twenty-three. So young with so much more in front of her. It didn't seem fair. I experienced a number of different emotions as I began to grieve.

Mum and dad and the rest of the family and friends offered their support after hearing the tragic news. I couldn't believe it was happening. After everything I had been through, the person who had supported me most and given her love and looked after me through hard times was gone. I found myself in a difficult situation as I had never been introduced to Eva's family and once again because of the language barrier it was going to be difficult for me to be able to express my feelings. It would have been hard enough in English, let alone in my basic Spanish.

I had some of Eva's friends come around to visit me and offer their condolences. As some of Eva's friends were Spanish I decided we would phone her family in Spain and try to express our sympathies. We rang the number that I had been given by Eva, and one of our friends, Raphael, conveyed how we were feeling to her mum and Dad. I spoke to some of Eva's friends in Spain that could speak English and was told how terrible they were all feeling. It was custom in Spain to have the funeral the next day, so I was told by the different friends that I spoke to that they would buy some flowers for me with a message to lay on her grave.

Because I wasn't able to attend the funeral, it didn't really seem real to me. I somehow expected to have the phone ring and hear Eva's cheerful, happy voice on the other end of the line. But the more time went by, the more it sunk in that she was gone. I cried in bed at night as I tried to come to terms with everything that had happened. It was at this time that I began to question my new-found faith. I noticed I was becoming cynical and bitter, something I told myself I didn't want to become. My mum was particularly worried that the grief would somehow trigger another psychotic episode. By this stage, I had stopped taking the medicine prescribed as the psychiatrist was of the impression that I would not encounter any more problems.

My life seemed once again to be in disarray and my future was unsure. I still had the plane ticket for Spain but felt at that time that visiting Spain would cause more grief and a part of me was thinking it would probably be best not to go to Spain. I had been in contact with Steve who was also upset at the death of Eva. Even though I had only met Steve a few years previously while travelling in Europe, he felt like one of my closest friends. I told him I was feeling completely lost without Eva and that my plans for the future had been turned upside down.

After some consideration I decided to cash in my plane ticket for Spain. This decision had also been influenced by a conversation I had with Eva's mother. She had explained that it probably wouldn't be a good time to come over as the family was trying to deal with the grief. After a few more phone calls to Steve, who was now living in Melbourne, I felt it probably would be good for me to take a trip to Melbourne and take my mind off things. So, within a few weeks I told my family that I was going to go to Melbourne to catch up with friends and that it would give me a chance to think about my future a bit more.

It didn't take long before I had booked my flight to Melbourne and with only my backpack I was on my way. I hadn't been to Melbourne for a number of years and was looking forward to getting out of Perth and catching up with Steve and some of my other friends. I was picked up at the airport by Ashley, who had decided to move from Perth to Melbourne. I immediately felt I had made the right decision as we drove to Ashley's house from the airport. A change of scenery and the chance to see some of my friends that I hadn't seen for a while seemed like the right thing to do.

Within a few days of being in Melbourne I got to catch up with Steve. Steve was living in St. Kilda and asked if I wanted to stay with him and his brother for a week or so. I spoke about the tragedy with Steve, who had also become quite good friends with Eva in London. It was good to talk to Steve, I found him to be really helpful. He suggested it would probably be best if I tried to enjoy myself whilst I was in Melbourne rather than concentrating on Eva's death so much. So, with Steve, his brother Bruce and a few other friends I started going out and decided to put the tragedy to the back of my mind.

During my two weeks in Melbourne I tried to enjoy myself, almost putting on a front and burying the pain. I found that there was always something happening Melbourne, so my mind was always occupied. I still thought about Eva and thought how much she would have enjoyed Melbourne. I would occasionally talk about Eva with Steve and Bruce and they could detect that it had made me bitter. I wasn't denying the existence of a higher power but I was confused at the purpose of taking Eva's life at such a young age.

I often thought about Eva just prior to going to sleep at night. I would think about the times we would take walks through the park and talk philosophically about the whole mystery of life. I would think back to the times when we would talk about travelling again together. We always said how we would like to travel to South America at some time in the future. Eva shared my passion for life experiences and neither of us were too concerned with material possessions. We both saw life as one big adventure.

After spending two weeks in Melbourne, I had to think more about my future. I thought about Perth and what I had to go back to. I didn't have a job and besides my family and some friends I didn't feel I really had a lot to return to. I had enjoyed the time I spent in Melbourne and felt that I had more in common with my friends in Melbourne as we were all single. I thought that I could make Melbourne a new chapter in my life. I didn't need too much encouragement from my friends before I came to the final decision that I would stay.

I got in contact with my family and some friends in Perth and said I had made the decision to stay in Melbourne. They were all very supportive and mum and dad felt the change would be good for me.

So, with only my backpack full of clothes, I started to get myself set up. Steve and Bruce had said that I could stay with them until I had found a job and a place and was on my feet. Getting back on my feet was to prove more difficult than I first thought. I hadn't worked since before I was first hospitalised in Spain. I had to think about what I was going to do. My plans to teach English in Spain made me think about teaching English in Melbourne. The qualifications I had gained in England weren't recognised in Australia so this meant I was going to have to fall back on my experience in banking. I was very reluctant to work in banking again but I didn't have a great deal of money and was going to have to find work soon.

I had started doing some voluntary work at a primary school that Steve was working at part time. I was working afternoons at an after-school care centre with kids aged between 5 and 10 years old. It didn't take long before I was offered some part-time work. It really was a good job, which mainly consisted of playing football in the park or helping with painting and crafts whilst looking after the kids. I really enjoyed working with the kids and found it to be rewarding. I was earning enough money to get by and it allowed me to put off working in banking.

After being in Melbourne for a few months I found I was becoming more confident and finding myself returning to the way I had felt prior to the breakdown in Spain. I was going out a lot in St. Kilda, which was a fun place to be. I was going to a few of the pubs in St. Kilda that were in the middle of a number of travellers' hostels. I would quite often go out on my own as Steve and Bruce were both studying. I found I was able to put on a front which hid the turmoil I had experienced over the past few years. I enjoyed meeting travellers from all over the world and would share travel stories. It reminded me a lot of my time in London and the many interesting people I had met. Each night that I went out I would meet more travellers who shared the same outlook on life.

One night I met a young Spanish girl called Begona from San Sebastian in the north. It was a chance to practice the Spanish that I had been studying. I enjoyed Begona's company, she was very friendly and like Eva. I found talking to Begona brought back memories of Eva. Memories that I had tucked away in a corner of my mind. I was noticing that I was repressing a lot of the memories I had of Eva and continued to show a happier side of myself. I was drinking quite heavily during this period of time. I found the alcohol gave me the numbing effect that I needed.

I was still living with Steve and Bruce in their small flat. I spent most of the days sleeping before doing some work at the primary school and then returning to the bars again at night. I finally decided that I was going to have to find some more work. It didn't take long before I found some work in banking as a part-time customer service officer in a call centre not far from St. Kilda. I worked in the bank in the mornings and the primary school in the afternoons. I found I was enjoying my new life in Melbourne. I was able to bear working in a bank as it wasn't as stressful as other jobs I had done in the past, and I looked forward to the afternoon when I looked after the kids. It proved to be an interesting contrast. I would listen to people moaning and whingeing about their money and get a sense of the pressures of society, hearing the stress and worry in the voices of the customers. I would then walk across a park to be greeted by between twenty to thirty children, totally oblivious to the pressures of modern society, only concerned with if I could play cricket or football with them. I was content for the time being and I could see myself staying in Melbourne in the immediate future.

I became quite good friends with Begona and eventually told her about Eva and what had happened. She was understanding and proved to be a good person to talk to. Begona was living in one of the hostels in St. Kilda so it was a good chance to meet other travellers. One night I was introduced to an Irish girl called Aideen, who, as well as having attractive looks, possessed a bubbly personality. After talking to her briefly I became aware of her sharp, witty sense of humour. I couldn't believe the chemistry there was between us. We ended up spending the whole night together talking and laughing. I hadn't seriously thought about getting involved with anyone but I felt so comfortable talking to Aideen that I thought there might be a possibility. As it turned out, Aideen had a boyfriend so my hopes were deflated somewhat. After thinking about it I felt it was probably too early to get involved with someone in a relationship so soon after the death of

Eva. I continued to see Aideen as a friend although it was difficult as I was still feeling very attracted to her.

I continued to go out quite a lot in St. Kilda and just concentrated on enjoying myself. My mental health appeared to be good, although I was still drinking quite heavily. It's only now when I look back that I realize that I really was abusing my body during that time. I was constantly drinking with a number of different friends that I had made at the bank as well as a number of travellers I had met. I was caught up in the atmosphere and began to feel happy in the life I had created for myself in Melbourne. This party lifestyle continued over a number of months and at the time I felt I deserved to be enjoying myself after what I had been through over the previous few years. I was, however, burning the candle at both ends.

I continued to see Aideen during this time and we became quite good friends. The more I got to know Aideen the more I realised how similar we were. I was still attracted to her and it was after some six months that she told me she was having problems with her boyfriend. Aideen had been with her boyfriend Mark for ten years and she explained she had come out from Ireland with the intention of marrying him. She mentioned how things weren't working out. This news made me think about the possibility of something developing between us.

I was still very hesitant about getting involved in a relationship and although I felt comfortable with Aideen there were still a number of things about my past that I hadn't told her. I wasn't sure how she would react and I suppose at that time, as no final diagnosis had been made, I was still unsure of how to explain some of the things that had happened in the past.

As time went by and it became clear that there was a very real possibility of something developing between Aideen and I, I decided I would just let things happen naturally. I thought if it was meant to be it would work itself out. It wasn't too long before something did happen. Aideen and I went out one night for a few drinks as we had done on a number of occasions and this night it became quite clear that Aideen and Mark's relationship had broken down, and she was showing more interest than she had done in the past. Aideen ended up coming back to the house I was renting and as I expected things unfolded as I felt they were destined to. I was feeling happy yet apprehensive at getting involved with Aideen and as we talked about any sort of a future together Aideen was honest in saying that she still cared for Mark. I understood how she would still be feeling this way and we both agreed to take things slowly.

Over the course of the next few months things seemed to go anything but slowly as we spent a lot of time together. I still hadn't told Aideen about my past, I suppose I was still unsure of when the right time would be and exactly what I would tell her. As Aideen and I spent more and more time together and became closer, she could sense that there was something I wasn't telling her. I decided to tell her I had become ill in Spain and was later diagnosed with having a thrombosis. I decided not to tell her that I had been in the psychiatric ward of the hospital.

I found I was attracted to Aideen because, not unlike with Eva, we felt comfortable talking about spirituality. Aideen had been brought up as a Catholic but the thing I admired about her was that despite Catholicism being the dominant religion in her culture, she had chosen to view it objectively and had her own beliefs.

As time went by I found I was starting to fall in love with Aideen. I was happier than I had ever been before and my attempts to stop myself from falling in love seemed futile. I felt as though I was experiencing emotions that I had never experienced before as my happiness turned into euphoria. I didn't realise it at the time but I was manic. I was seeing the world though different eyes. Everything seemed to be surreal. My thoughts seemed to be surreal and were once again starting to race. As this was all happening I hadn't seen Aideen for a few days. I still hadn't told her about all of my past but I was sure that Aideen would understand. As my thoughts continued to race I found I was unable to sleep. I hadn't slept for two days and hadn't been to work. I was in a world of my own. I decided to ring my mum in Perth to try and share the happiness I was feeling. As I rang and began to talk to her she could sense that my happiness was not normal. She said that I was talking too fast as I spoke to her and that she was concerned about me. I told her about how I had fallen in love, and that was in my mind at the time the reason I was acting the way I was. She asked me why I wasn't at work as it was the middle of the day. I was confused as to why she wasn't sharing in my excitement and hung up, saying that I would be in contact again soon.

My mania soared as I began to lose touch with reality. The happiness I was feeling was overwhelming. I decided to walk to the beach and breathe in the fresh sea air. I wanted to share my excitement with someone and after going to the beach I decided to call around and see Bruce. I didn't realise it was still quite early when I arrived at Bruce's flat and rang the doorbell and woke him up. He came to the door and by this time I was feeling jubilant and eager to share the feeling. Bruce was a bit confused by the way I was acting and asked if I was feeling alright. Bruce thought I was high from smoking drugs and refused to believe me when I explained it was a natural high. Little did I know at the time that the mania I was experiencing was due to a chemical imbalance. I told Bruce how I hadn't slept for a few days because of the happiness I was experiencing. After talking to Bruce for an hour or so he explained that he was going to work. He told me to try to get some sleep as he left but I still found I was feeling too happy to sleep. After an hour of lying down I decided to try and contact Aideen. Because my thoughts were racing I was unable to remember her telephone number. The next thing I thought was that she might be at work. She was working in a restaurant in St. Kilda so I decided to go to the restaurant on the chance that she would be working.

I made my way to the restaurant hoping to see Aideen. I hadn't seen her for a few days and was looking forward to seeing her. When I arrived at the restaurant I was relieved to see Aideen serving some customers and found it hard to contain the joy I was feeling. She saw me and looked somewhat surprised and then made her way over to where I was standing. She asked me what I was doing and why I wasn't at work. I found that as I began to speak, just like my thoughts were racing, it difficult to control the speed that I was talking at. I told her how something was happening to me that I couldn't explain and that I was happier than I had ever been before. She looked confused by the way I was acting and my mood continued to soar as I continued talking. By this time we had walked outside the restaurant and I couldn't control how happy I was feeling as I became euphoric explaining how I had fallen in love with her. Aideen still seemed confused by my behaviour and she eventually said that I should try to calm down and get some rest as she could tell by my appearance that I hadn't slept for a few days.

I left Aideen still feeling on a high and rather than going home thought I would go into the child care centre and explain why I hadn't been at work for a few days. I caught a tram to the primary school and as I walked towards the school I saw the children playing in the park. I began to notice how lethargic I now was feeling and knew that I wouldn't be able to work. I went into the centre and, after trying to compose myself, explained to one of the assistants that I hadn't been feeling too well and that I wouldn't be able to come in for a few days. I then decided to return home and try to get some rest. I became very tired as I walked and my mood had begun to change. I started thinking about my behaviour when I saw Aideen and how it must have been very confusing for her. I was beginning to regret that I had visited Aideen in the state that I was in. I started to become depressed and worried that my behaviour had scared her off. I became more and more depressed. My mood had changed completely from the way I had been feeling over the previous few days.

I eventually made my way back to the house where I was living. When I arrived I went to lie down on the bed and I wrestled with my feelings. I felt completely empty as I lay on the bed contemplating what I would do next. I was so tired, yet my mind was still racing and I couldn't get to sleep. After an hour or so the phone rang. As I picked up the receiver I heard Aideen's voice. She was asking if I was alright. She then said she was going to come around to visit me. Once again my mood began to lift as I became excited at the prospect of seeing Aideen again. I was trying to remain composed and when she eventually arrived I tried to act as normal as I could. Aideen then asked me what was happening and said that she was worried by my behaviour. I explained that I had experienced psychiatric problems in the past and that something had been happening to me over the past few days. I thought it might be a good idea to get in contact with the hospital so that I could talk to a psychiatrist. Aideen rang and tried to explain what had happened and I then explained that I hadn't been feeling well. The doctor thought it would be best if I went to the hospital for a further examination. I apologised to Aideen for everything and explained how I felt talking to a doctor would help.

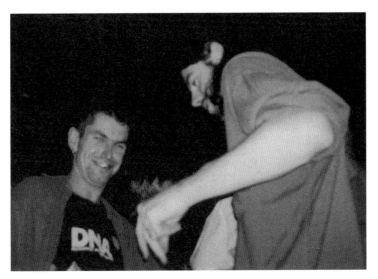

Bruce and Steve Carroll

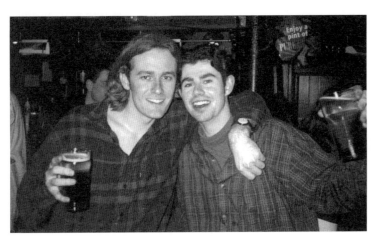

Enjoying a beer at the pub with Steve

6

Relapse

I arrived at the hospital still feeling as though my thoughts were racing and I was trying to gain control and remain calm. I was feeling extremely tired from not having slept for a number of days. I was registered as a patient and was told to wait until a doctor was able to see me. I waited with Aideen in a small waiting room with a few other patients. It felt like I had to wait for about an hour or so and I was becoming more and more tired and was frustrated that I couldn't sleep because of the racing thoughts. Eventually a female doctor came into the waiting room to talk to me and she asked me to explain what had been happening over the past few days. I mentioned how my mood had been up and down and that I was tired from a few days without sleep. The doctor was helpful and explained that I would need to spend a few days in hospital so that I could be given some treatment.

I was told that I was going to have to be transported to the mental health campus in an ambulance. Aideen had been with me through the evening and by the time I had finished talking to the doctor it was around midnight. Aideen became quite upset; the stress of what had happened had gotten to her and she broke down crying as I got into the ambulance. I said I was sorry and that I appreciated her support.

I arrived at the mental health campus after an hour or so. A mental health nurse had a chat to me and I was given some sedatives to finally help me sleep. I awoke the next morning feeling refreshed after getting about ten hours' sleep. I went out into the dining area of the hospital and noticed that I was in an enclosed area of the hospital. My mood felt better and I wasn't experiencing racing thoughts. Actually, my mood had returned to be on a bit of a high. I spoke to a mental health nurse and was feeling quite coherent. I went for a walk outside into an enclosed courtyard area and wondered whether I was the only patient in the hospital. I felt I had so much energy, and I didn't like being trapped in a confined space. I walked around the courtyard a few times and then returned inside. As I went back inside I noticed a couple of other patients sitting down having breakfast. There was a guy and a girl, both about my age, and they both didn't look well. They looked as though they were fighting depression. The girl looked like she had a tonne of weight on her as one of the nurses was talking to her, trying to help her. The guy was experiencing a few problems also and I was sensing that I should stay away from him and let him deal with his problems.

I went back to my room and had a lie down and that afternoon I was told I had a visitor. It was Bruce, who came in to see if I was alright. He said Aideen had called him to let him know I was in hospital. Bruce was concerned about me and hadn't known how bad I had become after I had left his place the previous day. Bruce brought me some music and a walkman to help pass the time. I explained how I didn't like being in an enclosed area and that I was looking forward to talking to the doctor so that I could hopefully go out to the open ward. Bruce left after spending a few hours with me and said he would come back to visit me again.

Later that afternoon Aideen came to visit me as well. I said

I was feeling better and that I was hoping to get out as soon as possible. I felt like I was still on a bit of a high and at the time didn't really accept that there was obviously something not right. I was still in a state of denial and when I spoke to the doctors and nurses explained that I didn't really feel there was anything wrong with me. This was influenced by the way I was feeling at the time and the frustration I was feeling at being in an enclosed area. The doctors that I spoke to felt that I was coherent and allowed me to go to the open ward, saying that I would be re-assessed the next day.

In the open ward I interacted with a few other patients. I remember there was a piano in the ward and a few of the patients would play piano which proved to be quite soothing. There was one girl that I talked to who seemed quite nice and she asked me to come into her room as she had some paintings she wanted to show me. I was amazed at how talented she was and she explained that she had been diagnosed with bipolar disorder but actually felt that her manic phases helped her to be more creative.

The next day I spoke to the doctor and nurse and once again explained that I was feeling fine and that I felt there was a spiritual component, as some of my experiences had made me more spiritually aware. I was instructed to go back onto the medication I had previously taken. But upon my release I didn't continue taking the medication and I only now realise that I was in denial. At the time I felt I could control my mind and didn't need the medication.

Bruce and Aideen picked me up from the hospital and I got home and slept again that night. When I woke the next day I felt like getting away for a few days on my own and reflecting on what I had been through. I went down to Lorne just south of Melbourne and stayed in a backpackers place on the beach. I spent a few days lying on the beach and going for bushwalks with some of the travellers I met at the hostel. I still felt on a bit of a high and didn't realise at the time that there was still an imbalance in chemistry in my brain, with an increase in serotonin. I loved the feeling of being on a high, which probably was why I didn't want to take any medication that was going to take away my highs. After a few days in Lorne I returned to Melbourne. When I arrived home Aideen called and said that she had been worried about me as she hadn't heard from me for a few days. I apologised and just said that I needed to get away from Melbourne. I said that I would catch up with her in the next couple of days. Later that night I got a phone call from the after-school care centre coordinator, explaining that she was short-staffed and asking if I could come in and help her out. I had already told the bank that I was unwell the week before and I was going to have to get in contact with them to let them know how I was feeling.

I went into the school the next day and helped look after the kids which I thought was the right thing to do. Unfortunately it turned out to be a typical Melbourne day with quite a bit of rain. This meant I had to get between thirty and forty kids inside, out of the rain. I hadn't anticipated how stressful this would prove to be. Screaming kids within an enclosed area and thunder and rain outside proved to be very stressful and I could feel that my mind still felt somewhat fragile from everything I had been through. I somehow managed to get through the day and looked after the kids with the help of the coordinator until their parents picked them up. After the last child had gone I explained to the coordinator that I still wasn't feeling well and was going to need time off. She understood and agreed to give me some time off.

That night I met up with Aideen and explained I still wasn't feeling one hundred percent. I then asked if Aideen wanted to come away with me as I had enjoyed the few days I had spent in Lorne. Eventually I talked her into coming down to Lorne with me. We had a good couple of days away. It also gave us a chance to talk about our relationship and where it was heading. Everything seemed to be happening so quickly in our relationship and I suppose I was a bit unsure at what the future would hold for us.

Aideen explained how she had to make some big decisions about her future. She was honest in saying that she still had feelings for Mark but at the same time cared about me. After a few days in Lorne we returned to Melbourne, with me still unsure of where our relationship was going. I started to think about what I was going to do as I really cared about Aideen but I didn't have any control over the destiny of our relationship. I started thinking that with all the health problems I had encountered once again and the uncertain future of the relationship it would probably be a good idea to head home to Perth and give myself a chance to think about what I was going to do.

Within a few days I had decided and I told my friends that I was going back to Perth. I hadn't told Aideen yet but decided that before I was going to tell her I would make one last effort to show her how much I cared about her. In the week before I was planning on leaving it was Valentine's Day. I thought what better opportunity than on Valentine's Day? I planned a surprise picnic in a local park. There was a show there afterwards by the state orchestra and in another part of the park there was a Shakespeare play. I organised the picnic and surprised Aideen with a rose. I was trying everything to show her how much I cared. She was impressed by my attempt at romance and later came back to my house where I had said there were another ten long-stemmed roses waiting for her. After a great night I told her of my plans to head back to Perth. She was shocked when I told her but I explained that I needed to go back and sort myself out and I wanted to see my family. Aideen said that she could understand and said she would get in contact with me after I arrived in Perth.

7

Return to Spain

I arrived back in Perth within a couple of days of resigning from my jobs and saying goodbye to Aideen and the friends I had made in Melbourne. I was picked up at the airport by my brother Andrew who I had earlier called and we had organised to make it a surprise for mum and dad. I was looking forward to seeing mum and dad as I hadn't seen them for a year. I had called mum to try and explain my previous phone call which must have been confusing for her. Looking back now, I think a lot of the time before I was diagnosed with an illness must have been confusing for mum and dad, particularly my erratic behaviour.

I arrived at the house and knocked on the door. The look on my dad's face was one of shock and surprise. I gave him a hug. Mum, who was equally surprised, was glad to see me. I chatted to them and said I was going to give myself a bit of time to think about my future as a lot had happened in the past year. I told them I had met Aideen and wasn't sure what the future would hold. I said it was quite a confusing time for me as I was still thinking about Eva and felt I wanted to go to Spain to give me some closure. I explained Aideen's visa was expiring soon and there was a possibility I could be heading over to Ireland. My future seemed to be up in the air as I hadn't anticipated meeting Aideen so soon after Eva's death.

Mum and dad were concerned about my health and asked if I could visit the doctor and explain how I had been feeling. The fact that I had been on such a high and actually feeling quite good added to the denial I was experiencing.

For the first few weeks back in Perth I caught up with some of my good friends and just relaxed after a year of working. It wasn't long before I heard from Aideen and she said that she had been thinking about me and was planning on coming to Perth before travelling through Asia on her way back to Ireland. I was having to make some decisions about my future and what I was going to do once again. I started thinking about how complicated I had made my life by falling for foreign girls. I told Aideen that I had been thinking about her too and that I had thought about going to Spain before meeting up with her in Ireland. She thought it sounded like a good plan and we could discuss it further when she arrived in Perth.

I told my parents of my plans and they were concerned about my health first and foremost. I had been to see a doctor as they had wished, but looking back I probably wasn't as truthful about my condition as I should have been. I would simply say that I was on a bit of a high and sometimes experienced dark thoughts but that I was feeling good. I had explained I was finding it hard to sleep and I had had some sleeping tablets prescribed for me.

Aideen arrived a month after I had left Melbourne and I was glad to see her. I definitely had very strong feelings for this girl. I found I was really comfortable with her and was starting to think maybe this was the girl for me. During the time she was in Perth I took her to the usual tourist spots and we had nice times.

We talked about the future and the prospect of me living in Ireland for a while. I was on such a high at the time and felt as though there was a future for us. I explained it was important for me to go to Spain to visit Eva's grave so we talked about possibly meeting in Spain for a brief time before heading to Ireland. Aideen had already planned a three-month trip through Asia so I thought I would go to Spain for the three months that she was travelling through Asia. I thought I could pick up some work in a bar for the summer which would give me a chance to practise my Spanish. Aideen said she was going to Bali for a few weeks before she headed through Indonesia, Singapore and Malaysia. Eventually I decided to spend a couple of weeks with her in Bali before heading to Europe.

Mum and dad could see that my mind was set on going back to Europe with Aideen and that there wasn't a lot they were going to be able to do to stop me. They were naturally still concerned about my health and were worried that I would encounter more problems. It's only now that I realise I was being quite selfish and not taking into account the worry that I was causing. I certainly wasn't thinking rationally at the time as I was still on an emotional high from the mania I had experienced as well as from the way I felt about Aideen.

It wasn't too long before it was time for us to fly to Bali and the start of another adventure for me. We picked up our tickets and mum and dad somewhat reluctantly took us to the airport. The night before we had had a family dinner to say farewell and once again my brothers and my mum had said they were concerned given what had happened on my previous trip. I explained how I would be with Aideen for a part of the trip and I had friends that I would meet up with in Spain. I had also improved my Spanish quite a bit since the last time I was in Spain so I would be able to communicate more effectively if I encountered any problems. I remember trying to sound convincing and alleviate their concerns.

After Aideen and I arrived in Bali we made our way to Kuta beach where we stayed for a few days and just relaxed. Afterwards we went up north and later to Lombok. We continued to enjoy each other's company, but after a couple of weeks together we started noticing things about each other we hadn't noticed before. We came to realize that we were both quite strong-minded, and we would argue our point strongly if we disagreed on something. After just over a couple of weeks we made our way back to Kuta as I was due to fly to London. We had enjoyed the time we had spent together but it had also made us aware that there were some differences between us.

I hadn't experienced any problems with my health apart from a touch of the famous "Bali Belly". My mental health had been good and I was now starting to look forward to heading back to Europe.

My flight to England was a morning flight and Aideen and I woke up early to have some breakfast before heading to the airport. I was concerned about Aideen travelling through Asia on her own and asked her to get in contact with me from time to time to make sure she was alright. I said my final goodbyes to Aideen at the airport and told her I was looking forward to seeing her in Spain in a few months.

I had organised to meet a friend, Gavin, at the airport in Barcelona and as I flew in over the Pyrenees Mountains I began to look forward to returning to Spain. Although I had some unpleasant memories of Spain from my previous trip I thought it would be good to get back and spend some time there.

I saw Gavin in the arrival lounge after passing through customs and we made our way to Blanes, a town just north of Barcelona. Gavin was actually a friend of my younger brother Cam and he was spending a few months in Blanes with another friend of Cam's who Cam had met while travelling in America, called Kevin.

Kevin was good enough to allow me to stay with him until I found some work. Blanes was a beautiful coastal town that was a popular tourist destination for British tourists. Kevin was working in a hotel and had a number of contacts around Blanes to help me find some work.

The first few weeks in Spain I spent my time with Gavin in and around Blanes. It was great to be able to use my Spanish which had improved markedly since my previous trip. I enjoyed meeting Spanish friends of Kevin's and went out to some of the restaurants and bars in the town. I found I was acting as an interpreter for Gavin as he wasn't able to speak Spanish. There were a couple of girls living in the house with Kevin who were unable to speak English so I found I was speaking quite a lot of Spanish. The improvement in my Spanish from when I had been in hospital in Spain gave me a lot of confidence.

My health since the time I had left Australia had been good, although I was still feeling on bit of a high. I got into contact with mum and dad to let them know I was fine and that I was looking for work in Spain. I wrote a letter to Aideen's parents in Ireland to introduce myself and give them details of how I could be contacted in Spain. I was missing Aideen quite a lot. During this period of time I was still feeling high on love, which was heightened by the mania I was experiencing. I actually consider myself quite lucky to have been able to experience such intense emotions, which for a normal, healthy mind are quite pleasant. I've been lucky enough to feel those strong emotions about ten times over. It really is an amazing experience to experience mania – the joy, the euphoria. It's just unfortunate that the more the mania increases the more you begin to lose touch with reality. I have never taken any hard drugs but I can imagine the rush some people experience and why they become addicted. When you experience mania it is an escape from the everyday reality that most people face.

As I thought about Aideen I was looking forward to talking to her and making sure she was safe and well. After a couple of weeks in Blanes enjoying myself I knew that I was going to have to find work soon as I didn't have a great deal of money. I eventually was offered a job working in a bar overlooking the beach. The manager wanted me to work on the terrace so that I could use my Spanish to help with taking orders. It was a great job working in the bar at night and on the terrace during the day. I was working with a nice Spanish girl who had been working in Blanes for a number of years and she made me feel welcome. I had the intention of working for the summer and then meeting up with Aideen in Ireland. I had already organised to visit Elizondo at the end of the summer to visit Eva's grave.

During this whole period I had somehow tried to block out the tragedy of Eva's death. I really hadn't dealt with it very well. I really didn't know what I was supposed to do in terms of dealing with the grief. I didn't like how the grief had made me bitter and angry. I still think now of how tragic it was for Eva to lose her life. It still doesn't seem real, it doesn't seem fair.

I was trying to just concentrate on the positive feelings I was having and it was as though I had pushed the feelings of grief to the back of my mind. I was happy to be working again and earning some money. The manager of the bar said that he would be able to organise accommodation for me and put a lot of my pay away in an account for me. The first few days working at the bar were great and I really enjoyed seeing the customers and having a chat to the different tourists. There were quite a lot of British tourists and you would quite often get them requesting traditional English dishes, like it was a home-away-from-home for them. I also had a fair number of Spanish customers and it was great to be able to switch between the two languages.

Unfortunately, the fact that I was talking in two languages and was still quite high seemed to trigger my thoughts to begin racing again. It was as if my brain had been stimulated once again and because I was still partly in denial, I didn't have any medication to be able to stabilise my mood. I was starting to think about what I could do to try to gain control of my thoughts. When you have a mental illness you can be quite stubborn and think that you have control over your mind. Unfortunately, when your thoughts begin racing it's like trying to hold back a pack of wild horses. It is extremely difficult, yet because I had experienced psychotic and manic episodes previously it was as though I had some insight into what occurs.

I found after a couple of days working that I was very tired, yet once again unable to sleep. I still had the sleeping tablets that had been prescribed for me and decided after lying in bed for a few hours trying to get to sleep that I would have to take some. I took three sleeping tablets to help me get some sleep, yet the more the hours passed the more I couldn't sleep. I was becoming frustrated, as I knew that I was going to have to go to work within a few hours. I decided to get up and have a chat to the two Spanish girls sharing the house and explain how frustrated I was feeling. It was just as it had been in Melbourne during a previous manic episode, where my brain seemingly goes into overload, and three sleeping tablets didn't have any effect.

I went out for a walk at about three a.m. to try and clear my head, but as time passed by I found I was still unable to sleep. I just wanted to get a few hours to help me get through the day at work. I was getting more and more frustrated as I didn't want to miss work after just starting the job. Still, the hours passed by and before too long the sun began to rise as the new day arrived. I had now gone without sleep for over 24 hours. I went into the kitchen and thought about what I was going to do. I decided I should go into work and see how I'd go. Before I went to work I had to meet another one of the bar's employees who was from Scotland and needed help with some interpreting to renew his work visa. I met him outside the office and had a chat to him and found I was feeling very lethargic. He was a nice guy from Glasgow and he had a particularly strong Glaswegian accent. It was quite funny when I was doing the interpreting with the Spanish immigration officer as I was finding it easier to understand Spanish than the Scottish accent.

After helping the Scotsman renew his visa we walked along the beachfront to the pub where I was working. My thoughts didn't appear to be racing as they had done the previous night but I was feeling dead on my feet. When I arrived at where I was working I greeted Gloria, the Spanish girl I was working with, and started to update the menu for the day. It was a beautiful day without a cloud in the sky and there were already a number of people walking up and down the terraces. I could tell that it was going to be a particularly busy day. We had about twelve tables out on the terrace and it was my responsibility to look after all the tables.

Within an hour or so quite a few of the tables were occupied and before I knew it I was heading back and forth with drink orders. There seemed to be more people than the other days I had worked and I was soon having to do two or three things at once as well as talking in Spanish and English, and, just as I feared, this triggered my thoughts to begin racing. Everything seemed to be speeding up around me. I was trying to pull the reigns back on those wild horses and gain control of my thoughts but I was finding it difficult. I figured I was going to have to say something to Gloria, but how could I explain what was happening to me? To get from the terrace to the pub I had to cross a road and because I wasn't concentrating I walked out in front of a car, which slammed on its brakes. I made my way into the pub and went into the toilet and tried to get my thoughts together. I didn't know what I was going to do. I couldn't go back out to the terrace. I had to do something. I eventually decided that I would explain to Gloria that I had been vomiting in the toilet and I wasn't feeling well. I didn't think she believed me but I wasn't sure how to explain what had been happening to me.

After convincing Gloria that I would have to go home I walked back along the terrace and felt relieved that I was on my way back to Kevin's house. My mood once again soared into mania and I was as high as a kite. I became disorientated on the way home as

I was once again in a world of my own.

When I eventually made my way back to Kevin's house I went into my bedroom and lay down on the bed, trying to get my thoughts together. I heard Kevin in his room and decided to tell him what had happened and wondered what I should do. After talking to Kevin I felt it would be best to get to a hospital and once again talk to a psychiatrist.

Kevin's girlfriend, Maria-José, drove me to a hospital just outside of Blanes and after a short wait I got to talk to a doctor. This time I was able to explain what had been happening to me, unlike a few years previously. The doctor prescribed me some Valium, as he felt it would calm me down and help me sleep. After being in a Spanish hospital once again I felt although I was able to communicate more effectively the language barrier would still prove to be an obstacle for me if I was to have ongoing treatment in Spain.

I was wondering what I should do upon returning home and after giving it some thought and talking to Kevin I decided I should get to Ireland, with the intention to eventually meet Aideen there. I reacted somewhat hastily and decided I would fly to Ireland as soon as possible because I had already experienced a nightmare in Spain. I just felt I had to leave.

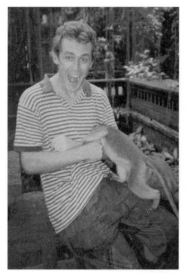
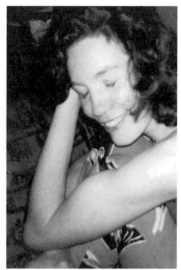

In Bali, with a monkey   *Aideen*

8

Ireland

Kevin felt that going to Ireland was my decision to make and as I was quite lucid, he agreed to drop me off at the train station. Before I knew it I had my bags packed and I was on my way back to Barcelona to head to the airport. I sat on the train as it made its way along the coast to Barcelona. I felt so tired but I could still feel my brain firing on all cylinders, even after a couple of Valiums and three sleeping tablets. My mind was still racing, yet not as much as it had whilst I was working. It was clear that stress seemed to trigger the racing thoughts. I had to change trains halfway down the coast and as I got off with my backpack my eyes felt very heavy, yet I knew that I wouldn't be able to sleep.

Whilst I was waiting for a connecting train I was wondering how I would make it to the airport without any sleep. If I could just sleep a few hours it would refresh me. I was sleep deprived yet couldn't do anything about it. I was lying down on my backpack, waiting for the next train, when I saw a hotel beyond the train lines. I thought 'if I could just get to a bed'. I got up and made my way towards the hotel but as I got closer I noticed that the hotel was looking out over a freeway on the other side. I kept walking and asked a group of people if they knew of another hotel in the area. I then walked up a laneway towards a small hotel that was hidden away from the traffic. I went into the reception and asked for a room. The lady behind the reception explained to me that there was a convention at the hotel and that there wasn't a single room available. I couldn't believe it. I walked down back under the underpass, feeling the weight of my backpack in my extremely tired legs. I made my way across to the beach and asked a group of young people if they knew where any other hotels were in the area. They said that besides the hotels that I had been to there was only one other, which had recently closed down.

I thought it obviously wasn't meant to be and that I should get on the next train and make my way to the airport. After another ten minutes or so the train for the airport arrived and I stayed on until I reached my destination.

I went up to the ticketing counter and asked for a flight to Ireland via London. I thought if I could get to Ireland I would then figure out what I could do whilst waiting for Aideen. I booked a flight to Cork in the south of Ireland as it was cheaper and shorter in duration. I didn't really know what I was doing but it just felt like getting out of Spain was the right thing to do. I boarded the plane and found my seat which was next to a window. I was still experiencing mania and was actually looking forward to the take off. I seemed to have some control over my mind and felt calm as a result of the Valium I had taken, as well as feeling high. As we taxied out onto the runway I fastened my seatbelt and was ready for what was going to be an amazing rush. As the plane picked up speed on the runway and began to take off it literally felt like I was flying, it was incredible. I looked out the window and enjoyed the experience. I looked back at Spain during the flight as we took the same flight path as my previous flight over the Pyrenees Mountains. It was a beautiful sight and I felt a sense of relief as I left Spain.

It wasn't too long before I landed at Heathrow airport in

London. I thought about staying in London but felt it would be best to head on to Ireland. I transferred flights and soon I was once again experiencing the rush of a plane taking off. We flew into the Emerald Isle in the early evening and although I was tired and still unable to sleep, I was looking forward to getting to Ireland, as I hadn't been there before.

The weather was quite overcast and there was a chill in the air as I disembarked and walked across the tarmac. I walked into the terminal, somehow dragging my legs under me, and made my way towards customs. I think the customs officer must have thought I looked suspicious as he stopped me with my passport to check I was the owner.

After making my way through customs I collected my backpack and then tried to organise some accommodation. I rang a few places but wasn't having any luck. I went out to the front of the terminal and jumped into a waiting taxi. I asked the driver to take me to a youth hostel. He said that it was a long weekend and as I had arrived on a Saturday it would be difficult to get accommodation. I was wondering when I was ever going to get to a bed.

The taxi driver dropped me off in the middle of Cork. Because I had arrived at night it made it difficult to try to orientate myself in and around the city. I went into the local youth hostel and noticed that there were a number of backpackers looking to check in. I got to the counter and was disappointed to find that the hostel was full. I then walked along a street filled with motels and bed & breakfasts and once again found that there were 'no vacancy' signs on the windows.

Because I had made the decision to come to Ireland somewhat hastily I didn't have a Lonely Planet travel guide or a map to help me find my way around Cork. I continued to walk around with my backpack on and my legs felt hollow by this point. I was becoming increasingly frustrated at not finding any accommodation. It was about nine p.m. by this time and I was starting to wonder what I was going to do. I spoke to a couple of guys sitting outside a shop and asked if they knew any other accommodation areas. They spoke with a broad Cork accent and pointed in the direction of a pub where they had rooms a few streets away. I walked up a hill and past a park and by this stage was contemplating sleeping in the park. I was wondering how I would go sleeping out in what had become quite a cold night. I decided to walk up towards the pub and try my luck.

I walked into the pub and took my backpack off and noticed that it was quite crowded, still everyone seemed to notice me walk into the pub. I could hear a band playing Irish folk music and a number of people enjoying themselves. I went up to the bar and asked if there were any rooms available and the barman shook his head. I had had just about enough by this stage and thought I would make one last effort to look through the phone book. I dialled a random number hoping to find a room available and decided if I didn't have any luck I would sleep in the park. Luckily for me someone hadn't shown up and the guy that answered the phone said I could have the room if I could get there in the next ten minutes. I asked him to hold it for me and after putting down the phone grabbed my pack and somehow forced myself to jog down the road. I waved down a taxi and asked him to take me to the address I was given as quick as he could.

I arrived at the motel within ten minutes and decided to stay a couple of nights and paid for it on my visa card. I made my way up to my room and let out a sigh of relief when I saw the comfortable bed. I made myself a cup of tea to warm myself up and then had a hot shower. I took another couple of Valium tablets and felt relaxed and was ready to have a long sleep.

I was amazed to find after a couple of hours of lying in bed and two days without sleep that I still couldn't manage to sleep. I eventually got to doze for a couple of hours before the effects of the Valium wore off. It was about 6.00a.m. Sunday morning and I decided to go downstairs to see when breakfast would be served. Everything seemed to be locked up in the dining area and there weren't any staff around. I went back to my room and had another shower. I watched a bit of the local television before returning to the dining room at around 8.00a.m. to have a traditional Irish breakfast.

I could feel the effects of the lack of sleep and the episode I had experienced in Spain, and as a result didn't feel totally coherent when the staff were talking to me. I look back now and realise I should have gone to hospital for further treatment.

I decided to go for a walk around Cork to try to orientate myself in the daylight. It was a beautiful day with a blue sky overhead. It seemed like a really nice place as I walked around. I found my memory was affected by the recent episode and I was having to constantly check to ensure I didn't get lost. I walked through a park not far from my motel and spoke to two young Irish girls. I asked them what there was to do in Cork on a Sunday. They said they were on their way to church.

We walked a fair distance across the park and through the centre of Cork. The girls were both university students and we chatted along the way whilst I took in everything around me. Cork was not unlike some English cities I had visited with older style buildings and streets. We continued walking towards a river that ran through the centre of Cork and crossed a bridge which led up to the church.

I thought going to a Catholic church in Ireland would be an interesting cultural experience and decided to go along with an open mind. I think the fact that during my manic state my spiritual beliefs intensified made me curious to attend church that morning. I was introduced to some of the girls' friends upon arriving at the church and found that the church filled up pretty quickly.

The minister began the sermon by reciting a number of prayers and I must have made it noticeable that I wasn't following as one of the girls alongside of me pointed to a passage in the bible. I continued to listen with an open mind but because I haven't had a particularly religious upbringing I was finding a lot of it quite foreign to me. I tried to fit in as best I could out of respect, but, as was the case when I was manic, I was thinking more philosophically during the sermon and viewed what I was hearing objectively. I suppose I've always been one to question what I am being told and I had the impression that the majority of people in the church, including the minister, only really thought one way and didn't think outside the square.

After the service I was introduced to the minister and because of my state of mind at that point I tried to put my viewpoint across that although I had a belief in a higher power I wasn't too sure about everything he had mentioned in his sermon. We then got into a theological discussion, with him trying to prove to me that everything he believed was true. I found he was adamant and unwilling to accept any other views than those he had been taught. He ended giving me a book to explain more about his faith and invited me back for a discussion later that night.

As I left the church after saying goodbye to the girls, I found that although I was somewhat sceptical I did have a feeling of calmness come over me as I walked down the street and back through the centre of town. The anxiety I had been experiencing appeared to disappear for a moment and my thinking became very clear. As I walked along the street I could hear singing in the distance and as I walked around the corner I saw a choir singing on the steps of a church. It was quite a beautiful sound but I noticed they were singing in a different language. As I stopped outside the church I asked a lady if she knew where they were from, she said they were Latvian Orthodox and were touring the country.

After stopping to listen to the choir I made my way to the park I had walked through earlier that morning. It really was a gorgeous day, with hundreds of people enjoying the sun. There were lots of families having picnics by a lake in the middle of the park. I spent some time lying in the park relaxing. I was still feeling very tired as a result of a lack of sleep. After an hour or so I headed off to get something to eat and had a brief walk around Cork before returning to my room. I decided I was going to head to the north as Aideen and I had discussed living in Galway when we had planned to go to Ireland.

That night I tried to sleep once again after taking a few more Valium tablets, but although I felt quite relaxed I wasn't able to sleep. I decided to read the booklet given to me by the minister earlier that morning at church. I found when reading it that the Catholic Church was trying to get people to follow its faith, but was doing this by trying to instil fear into anyone not choosing to become a Catholic by saying they'd be damned for eternity. I didn't think instilling fear into people was the right way to try and get people on board, or not for the right reasons anyway.

9

Mania and Depression

The next morning I had a shower and made myself a cup of tea. I once again barely got any sleep and because I was thinking irrationally at the time, I didn't go to the hospital as I should have and caught the train heading north up towards Limerick. I realised after boarding the train that I didn't have any money on me, so I got off the train at a small village called Mallow. I found an ATM after being given directions by a local. It was a really nice little town with only a few shops and houses surrounded by green fields.

Because I was disoriented I got lost on my way back to the train station and considered hitching when I found a main road leading to Limerick. Rain was beginning to fall and my attempts to get a lift were unsuccessful. So I eventually retraced my steps and got back to the train station.

Before too long I was back on the train to Limerick and trying to find some accommodation so I could get some more sleep. I was exhausted by this stage after going so long without a good night's sleep. I found a hostel not far from the train station in Limerick which was a bit cheaper than a bed & breakfast. I then lay down and drifted in and out of sleep until I eventually woke up in the early hours of the morning. I think the effect of lack of proper sleep and the imbalance of chemistry in my brain triggered another manic episode. I walked across the road from the hostel and felt totally disoriented to the point where I didn't know where I was and what I was doing there. I became higher and higher to the point where I was hypermanic, as was later described by a doctor. I found myself returning across a road near the train station and because I looked so disoriented I was apprehended by the police*. The police couldn't get any sense out of me and assumed I was on ecstasy because of my behaviour. They eventually took me to the police station for questioning and as my mania settled I explained that I had a history of mental illness and asked to see a doctor. Whilst I was waiting to see a doctor, immigration officers came to see me and asked where I was staying. They went to the hostel to pick up my things and confiscated my passports.

When the doctor arrived I said I wasn't sure what had happened to me over the past week and explained how I had had problems with my mental health in the past. He got me to sign a voluntary admission form and I was taken to hospital. After being taken to hospital I was given injections to help me sleep.

I awoke in a room with four beds, dressed in a pair of pyjamas and for a while wondering how I got there. Not long after I woke up a nurse came in and said I had slept for nearly two days and that I was only given sedatives until the doctor could talk to me. To my surprise as I walked out into the corridor Gavin was there waiting to see me. He said my brother Cam had contacted him to say I was in hospital. I worked out that they got my parents' phone number from my passport emergency numbers. I felt terrible, as my family all thought this would happen and I had been selfish and had gone ahead without seeing the consequences. I wrote

---

* The family felt an explanatory note was necessary here; Jamie's brother Andrew spoke to an Irish doctor after Jamie's arrest and was told Jamie had been arrested because he was directing traffic.

a letter, apologising for putting them through more worry and said I was feeling better and was going to spend some time in hospital getting treatment, and conceded that I obviously had a problem and was going to need help. After writing the letter and spending some time with Gav I went in to see the doctor. I tried to explain how I had been feeling prior to being brought into the hospital and he asked me if I had been taking any drugs as the police suspected. I said I hadn't and it made realise that perhaps the police don't have the appropriate training to deal with someone with a mental illness as they had assumed I was taking drugs and not that my behaviour could have been due to mental illness.

I spent about an hour talking to the doctor and he checked with a couple of hospitals in Perth to try to help him make a diagnosis. He said it sounded very much like I had had a hypermanic episode. I explained what had happened in Spain a few years prior and how the episode was similar although I didn't have the perception of hearing voices. The doctor, who was a very quiet-spoken man with a nice manner, assured me that he would be able to help me but that I would have to accept that I had a problem. He detected by talking to me that I was still in denial. He asked me what my plans were and I told him about my plan to meet up with Aideen after her trip. He urged me to return to Australia to get ongoing treatment. I was reluctant to return to Australia as I was looking forward to seeing Aideen again, but after giving it some thought I decided it would be best to return.

I told Gav I was going to go back to Australia but was going to explain myself to immigration first to try and get back my passports. Gav and I went along to the immigration office for a meeting and I explained how my behaviour was beyond my control and that the doctor's diagnosis supported that. To my relief I was given back my passports and before long I was discharged from hospital with enough medication for until I got back to Australia. I had been prescribed mood stabilisers (Resperidal) and found I was sleeping quite well once again.

Gav and I caught a flight to London and I thanked him for coming from Spain as I boarded my flight back to Australia. I took my medication as prescribed and found I got some sleep on the flight back. Gav rang my family to let them know I was coming home and what time I was due to arrive. After a stopover in Singapore the plane landed in Perth in the early evening. I wasn't too sure who would be at the airport and still felt bad at the worry I'd caused. As I got off the plane and walked through the departure gates I saw the whole family waiting for me. I was pleased to see them and gave Cam a birthday present I had bought in Singapore. I was relieved to be home and glad that things hadn't been worse.

The next day, after a good night's sleep at mum and dad's house, I went up to the hospital and got more medication. I made an appointment to see the doctor to get more treatment. I decided to see the doctor on a weekly basis until I was able to understand more about my illness.

After about a week of being back in Australia there was a phone call from Aideen, wanting to know where I was. Dad answered the phone and explained how I had returned to Australia because of my health. She was obviously concerned and was as disappointed as I was. I explained how I had a return ticket to the UK and would see how my treatment went before deciding to return.

Over the next few months I saw the doctor and gradually learnt more about the illness that he was sure was bipolar disorder. I worked part-time in a couple of temp jobs in administration type work but I as a result of everything I had been through I found it difficult coping with stress. I then did some labouring work with my dad who was doing some painting and decorating. I continued to keep in touch with Aideen by email and letters. I was missing her although time made me realise that I hadn't really dealt with

Eva's death very well. Over this period of time I was trying to deal with a kind of delayed grief, as well as coming down from the mania and going through depression. I found I was becoming more and more withdrawn and negative. I felt I was trapped in a dark room with no way of getting out. My parents were worried about me but I felt there was nothing I could do about it. After six months of not seeing Aideen and trying to continue a long-distance relationship I think she could sense that I still had a number of issues that I had to deal with and that it would be best to go our own ways. This saw me reach rock-bottom as I was probably using Aideen for emotional support. My depression seemed to be spiralling out of control and my parents rang the hospital to have me admitted.

I felt completely hopeless as I lay on the hospital bed, to the point where I found everything I had to deal with had gotten on top of me. I didn't see a way out of that dark room. My mum was looking into my eyes, telling me I was going to get through and not to give up. I felt lifeless as I lay staring at the ceiling, just feeling a kind of dull pain. The nurses had me on thirty minute observations and the doctor prescribed anti-depressants for me.

After about a week I started to feel a bit better and that dark room I felt trapped in was letting in a bit of light. I started to eat more and interact with the other patients. My mum and dad and my brothers had been up to visit me a few times and were glad to see that I was improving. I was discharged to the open ward after a week and attended group counselling and took part in some occupational therapy and recreation. After two weeks I returned home and felt better with the help of the anti-depressants. I spent a bit of time at home thinking about what I was going to do as I had to think about my future on my own again. I thought it would be best to live in Perth where I had quite a good support network of family and friends. I wasn't too sure what I was going to do for employment in light of the fact that I had had problems with work associated with the illness. The first thing I decided to do was to go to Melbourne and catch up with Steve, Bruce, Ashley and some other friends and give myself a chance to think a bit.

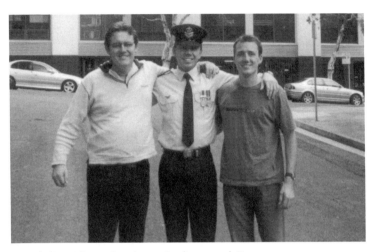

Me (left) with my brothers, Andrew and Cam

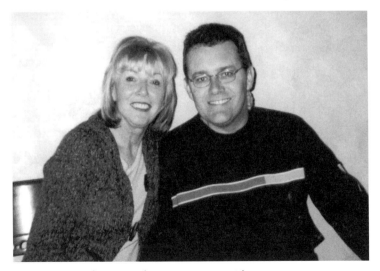

Having a meal in an Indian restaurant with mum

10

Opening a new door...

When I arrived back in Perth, after giving it some thought, I decided to continue studying. This was to gain more of an insight into my illness and gain qualifications that would enable me to eventually help people who have encountered similar problems. I enrolled in a Human Services Course at the local college to follow on from counselling and psychology that I had studied. I was due to start in the New Year, with the course lasting approximately a year.

I spent the holiday period with family and friends and found that I had begun to feel better after being hospitalised and given anti-depressants. I was looking forward to starting the course and meeting some new people as well as learning more about my illness.

I started the TAFE course in February and quite enjoyed being in a classroom situation once again after previously studying by correspondence. I met some nice people with similar interests and found my health to have improved. I managed to cope with the study but still found I could become quite tired mentally and wouldn't take on too much at once. I found the subjects to be interesting, as they covered a fairly broad spectrum, ranging from

Human Development, Psychology and Mental Health Issues to Human Rights.

I became quite good friends with one of the students who was my age. She had recently finished a relationship and we spent quite a bit of time together yet neither of us were really looking for another relationship. We helped each other with our studies and were more dedicated than some of the younger students. Margaret was interested in working in the outback as a Welfare Officer helping Aboriginal families. She was a very kind and caring person and always willing to help anyone out.

Whilst I studied I still enjoyed a social life with some of my friends in Perth, going out and having BBQ's. I also joined the local cricket club and became a bit more active as well as making new friends. I found that as more time went by I began to feel better within myself and learnt to cope with everything I had been challenged with.

I think that we are never given more than we can handle and within all of us is the strength to meet any challenge.

I could feel as though I had really grown as a person as a result of everything that had happened to me and that my life had presented challenges to enable me to grow. I found the journey of self-discovery that I had been on since the first episode in Spain had really allowed me to open up my mind. I felt as though I was racing down the freeway of life up to that point in Spain and after that I was forced onto a track that few have travelled before, that is a much more difficult path, yet a much more rewarding one. It was as if this track leads up a mountain looking over everyone who has continued down the freeway of life. It may be a harder road but the view is worth it.

I was starting to look inward for things to satisfy me rather than outward. Prior to leaving on my first world trip I was caught up in having material possessions and what society dictates, rather than trying to find peace within myself.

When I look back it was as if I was having to challenge everything that I had been taught and question things more to allow me to enter this door and try to find myself and the person I wanted to be. Although it may seem corny and clichéd, it really was a case of learning to love who you are, because I think you can start to find peace within yourself when you are comfortable with who you are as a person.

It was during this time that I started writing poetry and songs. I started writing songs with an old friend of mine, Steve, who is a singer/songwriter. I found it enabled me to express how I was feeling as well as giving me a sense of achievement hearing a song completed. Steve and I co-wrote a number of songs that we would play and sing when I would visit his house. He had quite a good set-up with production and sound equipment in his home studio. We would sometimes play and drink for hours until we were happy with the sound. Steve was a good singer and acoustic guitar player and between us we co-wrote seven songs on three CDs. Three of these songs were titled 'Out of the Cold', 'Guiding Light', and 'Heavy Soul'. Steve and I would go through periods where we wouldn't catch up for some time and other times where we would see each other weekly.

I also began writing this book as I felt it was a story that had to be told. I was hoping that people would be able to draw something from my experiences. I wanted to tell there is eventually light at the end of that dark tunnel. Writing notes for the book was also something that I would do over different periods where I felt motivated to get it finished. Sometimes it would go untouched for weeks without a single word being added because of the manic depression of bipolar. Yet other times I was so high being manic that I would just write and write pages of notes, some that I kept for this book.

After completing my TAFE studies I began working in an occupational rehabilitation centre known as Lorikeet House with people who have experienced psychological or psychiatric problems. The work generally consisted of helping people to develop their skills to enable them to re-enter the workforce. They would learn administration, computer and cooking skills in a supportive environment.

I started working at Lorikeet House for up to 40 hours a week. I'm not sure how it happened, but I found myself cooking lunch at the house for up to 30 people. I barely knew how to cook toast, and here I was cooking a range of meals for employees and patients. This continued for nearly three months and I was also helping with administration for Lorikeet staff while at the same time trying to cope with university study. I had been accepted to Edith Cowan University (ECU) as an undergraduate and had enrolled in 1st year Psychology, feeling this might help me further understand the way the mind works.

Apart from cooking, I found I was able to draw on my studies and helped a number of people at Lorikeet, which was rewarding although I found counselling to be quite difficult as I probably hadn't completely recovered from my own ordeal. I tried to help as best I could and found that I could empathise with people and their experiences. There came a point where I found the pace of the work and study too much to handle, so I decided to quit at Lorikeet and try and keep the study going. I also found this more and more demanding and stressful, so I had to withdraw and defer until another semester. In between re-enrolment at ECU, I attempted some voluntary work teaching migrants English. I had registered with an English school in Perth that was specifically set up to teach foreign students over a few months at a time. I had fun and met some interesting people, but again, I found I couldn't cope with the manic depression and the stress of teaching. In 2002 I re-enrolled at ECU in Sports and Marketing. This only lasted a few weeks before I had to withdraw for the last time.

I've realised from my time at Lorikeet that it is good to have support when you have experienced mental health problems but at the end of the day I think you have to learn to cope on your own. I think in a lot of ways you can be your own psychologist and help yourself because no-one knows you better. I also learned that I took on too much at once with work and study and that the bipolar was not going to let me cope with anything too demanding.

11

The puzzle

I believe that everything that has happened to me, happened for a reason. I feel as though I have changed as a result and that I may be well on the way to solving the puzzle.

Looking back I have come to the conclusion that the original breakdown was caused by insufficient rest after working long hours in London and triggered by alcohol at the festival. Even prior to the initial breakdown it was evident when I look back now that there were underlying problems. I think it was always going to happen, it was just a matter of time.

The psychotherapy I have had with Dr. Peter has helped me to cope with the illness although a lot about the illness remains a mystery. What really is Bipolar and can those diagnosed as having it all be placed into the same pigeon hole? Maybe this is just one way for society to accept and deal with mental illness.

When I look back over these years, there are a lot of gaps in the puzzle that psychotherapy hasn't been able to explain. I still haven't been given an answer as to how it was possible that my body was flung into the air when I was lying on the street in Spain. That was the defining moment in my life that was the start of a spiritual awakening for me.

Sydney 2003

Jamie suffered another severe manic episode in 2003. This is Cameron's account of what happened. Jamie wanted to have this included in the book.

Maaike and I moved to Sydney in February 2003 for my work. Jamie had planned to visit us after a visit to Melbourne to see his friends. It was just prior to Easter and Jamie was due to arrive that day.

I received a message on my mobile from Jamie, saying that he might not arrive on his intended flight as he was in the ER of a hospital waiting to see a doctor. He told me not to worry, that he was okay, but that he just had a few racing thoughts and that he thought it best to see a doctor. I rang him back and found his speech and thought process a little faster than normal. He did seem in control though. I was later brought up to speed by a friend of Jamie's and by the psychologist that Jamie spoke to. Both were comfortable that Jamie had caught his 'racing thoughts' in time and that he could still travel to Sydney instead of returning to Perth. I clearly remember the psychologist saying that Jamie seemed to have a good understanding of his illness and what triggers it and that he seemed to be in control. The psychologist in Melbourne prescribed Jamie some Valium to help him sleep and help him control his highs.

Jamie landed in Sydney the next day. I picked him up at

the Virgin Blue terminal. It wasn't cold, but Jamie was wearing several layers of clothing, including a large jacket… One very odd side effect of bipolar disorder seems to be that sufferers wear large amounts of clothing. Jamie was sitting with his bags, staring straight ahead with a strange smirk on his face. I gave him a hug. Jamie said: "I can see why some people take drugs like ecstasy. I'm just lucky that I can feel that way without the drugs." He was very obviously on a high.

Over the next few days, it was clear that Jamie was not the Jamie we know. He was more spiritual than normal, obsessed with intelligence and quite opinionated. He was also writing poetry and songs. His creative side was coming out more strongly. He would sing to Maaike and I a verse or two from some of the songs he'd written. The songs were spiritual, positive and often about love or surviving depression.

Despite taking the Valium to help him sleep, Jamie could only manage a few hours sleep before he was up listening to music and writing. It would be 4am and we would hear Jamie up and about trying to be quiet. The less sleep he had the more Jamie became 'wired' and his mind was clearly in a heightened state. He would become fixated with religion and try to relate it back to his own situation. Jamie felt that he was being punished for things that he done earlier in his life. Like one time Jamie had shot a bird when we lived in Sale - a country town in Victoria. He would almost be in tears explaining how bad he felt about what he had done.

Jamie was also preoccupied with what level of thinking others were on. He would ask what books Maaike had read and whether she believed in god. Maaike had studied history in the Netherlands and completed her thesis on the impact on society of Salman Rushdie's book *The Satanic Verses*. Jamie was fascinated by this, and believed that Maaike must be close to his level of thought.

The first few days were very tense and with Jamie getting little sleep we were all on edge. The doctor that Jamie saw in Melbourne recommended that we try to keep him calm and avoid over-stimulation. We took a nice walk through the botanical gardens and around the opera house. We attempted to grab a quick bite to eat in the city but the bustle of people shopping made Jamie more anxious. We went to a friend's barbeque and then decided to risk a football (soccer) game. It was after all supposed to be a holiday for Jamie. The Cronulla Sharks were playing Perth Glory in Cronulla. Maaike and I used to join Jamie watch the Glory play most games when we were living in Perth so we thought it would be like old times. One of my friends (Paul) decided to come along to watch the game as well after the barbeque.

The game was fairly uneventful until the last few minutes when Perth Glory scored the winner. Great for them, but it did get Jamie a little more worked up than what we had hoped. Interestingly, Jamie refused the cup of water Maaike had gotten him and went off to buy himself bottled water.

On the Monday night, Jamie was getting more worked up and I decided we couldn't wait until the morning to have him speak to a doctor. We phoned a psychologist on call and filled him in on Jamie's status. Jamie chatted with the psychologist and reassured him that he had it under control and that if he took a Valium he'd be okay to get through the night.

Around 10:30pm, Maaike and I were in bed chatting about Jamie's state of mind. We were both tired but finding it difficult to relax and get a good night's sleep. I got up to go to the toilet and say good night to Jamie. I asked him to not stay on the computer too long and keep the noise down as we had to work in the morning. Jamie asked if we could chat about a few things. We sat on the couch and Jamie proceeded to tell me about how he had found god and that if I opened up, I too could experience god. I reassured Jamie that it was great if that helped him to deal with things, but that I felt comfortable with my life and that if I was ever going through tough times I might look for something to help me through. Jamie then asked me if I knew what surreptitious meant. I wasn't 100% sure of the meaning. Jamie explained that it meant sneaky and said that he had heard surreptitious voices in the computer telling him to do things (maybe they were telling him to stay on-line; our next bill reflected that).

Worried about Jamie's state, I asked him to take some Valium so that he would get some sleep and then we could go to the doctor first thing in the morning. That's when I discovered Jamie did not have any Valium left. Okay that was it, time to seek professional help – tonight!

I called the on-call psychologist back and explained that Jamie was manic and needed help. Paranoia is another effect of mania, so Jamie followed me around so he could hear what I was saying to the doctor. Making sure I wasn't double-crossing him. I then passed the phone on to Jamie so the doctor could assess him. The psychologist had Jamie get his medication and explain the dosage and quantity he had. He then asked Jamie to remove one of the tablets that bring him down at night and take it while speaking on the phone. I stood next to Jamie and watched him take the tablet and make a swallowing noise for the doctor's benefit. Unfortunately Jamie then removed the tablet from his mouth and tried to conceal it. I said: "You have to take it Jamie." The psychologist could hear what was going on and also pressured Jamie to take it. That sent Jamie over the edge.

With his medication in one hand and the phone in the other, Jamie completely lost it. He started screaming "NOOOOO!" into the phone and hung up. His head started to shake and his speech was incoherent. It's hard to describe, but Jamie sounded like he was speaking backwards at various speeds. He sounded like someone else. He was hysterical, screaming, "I'm scared, I'm scared", knocking the bedside cabinet over as he lunged back into the bedroom wall. I managed to get him to lie down on the bed. He was disoriented and looked at me as if I was a stranger.

I tried to speak in a calm, reassuring voice, saying "It's me Jamie, it's your brother Cam, it's okay, you're safe." He kept wanting to leap off the bed so I restrained him by laying on him, rubbing his chest to try to calm him down.

Suddenly, the phone rang. It was the psychologist, asking me if everything was alright and wanting me to write down a number. So as not to make Jamie freak out again I said to the psychologist that Jamie 'was just a little worked up', and that I was calming him down. Of course my heart was leaping out of my chest, and I was wondering what the hell I was going to do! I couldn't write down the number the psychiatrist wanted to give me as I didn't dare take my hands off Jamie's chest, so I called out to Maaike, who had stayed in our bedroom (next to the one Jamie was staying in) to not aggravate the situation. Maaike came into the hallway and when Jamie noticed her, he screamed "You, You!" in a terrifying tone. Maaike quickly went back to our bedroom. I tried to calm Jamie, saying "it is only Maaike, you know Maaike Jamie". Jamie had no idea who she was, but he was terrified of her. I was relieved he recognised me. He'd say: "You're my brother Cam, I love you Cam."

Luckily, the psychiatrist had heard Jamie's violent outburst and had called the police. They arrived a few minutes later. As Jamie had directed his anger at Maaike, she decided not to risk going into the hallway and so climbed out of our bedroom window so she could explain the situation to the police. I asked Jamie to stay calm and stay in his bedroom so I could have a chat with the police. I assured Jamie that I had asked for them to be called and that they were here to help me, hoping that might work. I didn't want him restrained and arrested if I could help it.

I went out the front door and spoke to the police officer, I told him that Jamie had a mental illness, but that he trusted me and I could come with him to the hospital to keep him calm. By this stage, Jamie was standing calmly behind me greeting the policeman like nothing had happened. I told Jamie that we needed to get our shoes so we could go to the hospital. I told him the police were going to help by giving us a ride. I followed Jamie in to help him collect a few clothes. Jamie then whispered to me so the policeman couldn't hear: "Don't worry Cam, I'm not going to go with them." Great! Jamie then leapt onto the bed and started screaming again: "NOOOOO!" I jumped up and held onto him to try and calm him down. By now, four police officers were standing in the hallway ready to restrain Jamie. I kept saying: "It's okay Jamie, they are here for me, I called them." I managed to get him in the back of the police van and jumped in with him.

To distract Jamie, I very slowly tied up my shoelaces and helped him with his. I took as much time as I could, hoping the hospital was close by. Only 5 minutes later we arrived at Rozelle Psychiatric Hospital.

I was amazed at how calm the medical staff were. They said Jamie was the fifth admission for the night. They routinely commenced the paperwork necessary to have Jamie see the psychiatrist on call.

We were in the waiting room with the police watching on. By now Jamie was starting to try to explain his actions, as much for my benefit as that of the police. He mentioned that he felt he had been drugged by Maaike and my friend Paul at the soccer. He claimed they had spiked his water with cocaine. He said they couldn't be trusted. He apologised to me before saying: "I know she's your girlfriend and he's your friend Cam, but I think they drugged my water."

The psychiatrist went through some routine questions with Jamie like how he felt, his medical history and what happened tonight. Jamie predictably displayed calmness while explaining his illness and the medication he was on. I was thinking, please don't be fooled by this calm act…he needs help. The psychiatrist went to fetch some medication to help relax Jamie. I followed her to try to explain the real story. Of course Jamie thought I might try that and so followed me to hear what I was trying to say.

The psychiatrist asked a few more questions and Jamie finally displayed his paranoia. He looked at the tablets the psychiatrist provided and tried to read the writing on each tablet. He then looked at me to see if I trusted the doctor. I encouraged Jamie to take them. He then mentioned again about his water being drugged and that he couldn't trust Maaike. He said: "have you seen the books she reads? They're not right. She reads about satanic verses." I tried to reassure him that he misunderstood the title of Salman Rushdie's book. He didn't want to listen though as he wanted to place blame on others for his actions.

The psychiatrist could see Jamie was manic and paranoid and arranged for his admission to the general ward.

I remember the surprise of the psychologist in Melbourne when less than a week after he'd seen Jamie I contacted him to tell him Jamie had been admitted to Rozelle Psychiatric Hospital. He said, "I really thought he had it under control." One thing I've noticed about Jamie's illness is how good he is at manipulating people into believing he's okay. He says he's "just a little bit up at the moment." He clearly articulates his illness, history and medication needs, so most people (including many doctors) feel he has it under control. I've learned to see this as 'alarm-bell' time. I think he's actually trying to convince himself that he has it under control. With bipolar disorder, Jamie has experienced the lows of depression. So when he feels 'a little bit manic' he loves the happy feeling and wants it to be sustainable.

The next day I visited the hospital and asked to see Jamie. The nurse told me that Jamie had been transferred to the maximum-security ward, as he had tried to escape. The police were called and Jamie was found hiding without a shirt on in a creek at the bottom of the hospital gardens. His back was covered in mosquitos.

I called my eldest brother Andrew in Newcastle to explain what had happened. Maaike and I were completely drained and really needed a break. He said he would be down that night.

Andrew and I went to the hospital the next day. We felt it was too soon for Maaike to come just yet as Jamie had directed much of his anger at her. We went to the maximum-security ward and asked to see Jamie. In between the entrance and the actual ward is a small room with some couches where family and friends can visit the patients. Visitors enter through the front door while the door to the ward remains locked. When the front door is locked they then open the door to the ward to let the patient into the visiting area.

Jamie was standing at the door waiting for Andrew and me. He had all his belongings in his hands. When we asked why he had all his stuff with him, Jamie replied: "They said I'm okay to go. It's fine, we can go now." Andrew and I exchanged a look and then told Jamie that he needed to stay and that the doctors would have to decide when he was ready to go. Jamie got frustrated and felt that we had betrayed him. He said: "If you don't help me get out of here, I'm going to have to disown you as my brothers." Andrew and I couldn't help but smirk.

On other occasions, Jamie would come from behind the locked door carrying a bundle of literature. This was a mixture of brochures and papers about psychiatric help and the 'Intensive psychiatric care unit'. Jamie would continually refer to these 'books' as having the answers to the meaning of life, and told us that we should read them to find these answers.

Sometimes Jamie would just break down and cry during visits, without warning and for no apparent reason. Andrew or I would hold his hand and remind him that he was on the way to recovery, and that he would be ok. We kept reminding him that it would take time for the medication to start working. It was difficult for Jamie to be patient while in a manic state.

Jamie also claimed that he was now vegetarian. He didn't feel it was right to eat animals anymore. Knowing how much Jamie loves his meat and that he is not so keen on vegetables, we realised he was still a little way off from being released.

A couple of days later, Maaike came along to visit Jamie. All was fine; Jamie apologised for his actions and made light of it. When Maaike asked how the facilities were, Jamie replied: "People are a little bit confused in here. I try to help them where I can." Maaike is a vegetarian, so Jamie informed her that he now understood and agreed with her stance on not eating animals.

A few days had passed and the medication to bring down Jamie's mania was starting to take effect. We knew Jamie was getting better when he said he had had a sausage at a barbeque put on for the patients. He said the soy products and vegetables were not for him.

Jamie was released from the maximum-security ward to the general ward and was waiting for a final assessment from the doctor. Not long after that Jamie was released and back at our house. I had postponed his flight back to Perth and rescheduled his return for a couple of days later. Jamie was much better but still slightly manic. His conversations were still very spiritual but his medication had subdued his paranoia. Andrew returned to his work in Newcastle. I don't think we could have managed without him.

I drove Jamie to the airport and waited until he boarded his plane. When the cabin door closed I felt like a massive weight had been lifted off my shoulders. I felt like I could breathe again.

When Jamie is manic or paranoid I no longer see him as my brother Jamie. He's just someone that's sick and needs help. Anything he says or does is just a symptom of mental illness. I don't hold it against him. I just feel sad that he has to experience the mental pain of a breakdown. Unfortunately it's difficult to reason with him when he's manic, so we just help him through it. When he's more stable we talk about what happened and try to make light of it. With having to endure so much, I don't want Jamie to feel guilty or a burden on his family. We love him and will always support him.

Epilogue

As recounted in the previous chapter, Jamie was required to spend time in a mental hospital in Sydney in 2003, after experiencing another psychotic episode. After two weeks in Rozelle Psychiatric Hospital, Jamie was discharged to allow him to prepare to fly back to Perth for further treatment. A few days later, Jamie was again back in Perth with his parents and was required to undergo systematic therapy and a review of his medication, which was Epilim and Haloperidol.

Jamie continued to write his poems and work on this book, which he based on his travel diaries and scrapbooks that he had accumulated over the years. He had drafted notes for the last chapter just prior to Christmas 2003 and planned for the book to be transcribed before submission to a publishing company.

But Jamie's life was once again turned upside down on January 1, 2004. Jamie had just returned to his bedroom around 9 a.m. after getting out of bed to get a drink and wish his parents a 'Happy New Year'. A short while later, his mother discovered him collapsed on the bedroom floor. Jamie was rushed to hospital where he was diagnosed as having suffered a stroke. The stroke had caused an almost complete paralysis of the right side of his body and serious damage to parts of the brain. Jamie was unable to walk, communicate, eat, or drink. Tests and frequent consultations confirmed that Jamie had suffered a massive stroke, caused by a blood clot in his left carotid artery.

Jamie received intense therapy during 2004. Due to his age and strong will, Jamie managed to regain 90% of the strength and mobility that he had lost from the right side of his body. Jamie managed to regain control of some parts of the brain, which allowed him to resit his driver's licence. He passed. However, Jamie is still unable to communicate effectively and cannot write or think creatively, leaving him unable to write any more of his book, poems or music. Jamie has severe 'dysphasia'; his speech is very limited and he occasionally struggles to understand what is said. He continues to undergo speech and occupational therapy.

Jamie is now on a cocktail of medications to meet both mental health and post-stroke treatment. Further testing in 2004 revealed that Jamie suffers from the blood disorder known as 'Anticardiolipin antibody factor V Leiden'. This disorder relates to the increased likelihood of his blood clotting; increasing his chances of a further stroke. Doctors also discovered during earlier x-rays that Jamie had a growth on the left side of his neck, adjacent the carotid pulse. The growth was diagnosed as a benign tumour, but needed to be removed surgically before it grew too large and Jamie underwent surgery in early 2005.

The operation left Jamie with quite a scar; from the base of his left ear to the bottom of his neck (almost 6 inches!). Jamie's friends decided he deserved a get-well gift, one that would help him take his mind off all that he had been through. A week later, Jamie's friends had pooled their money and bought him a large flat-screen TV (see picture).

Jamie's family and friends have never ceased to be amazed at his will and determination. In the face of undeserved adversity, Jamie continues to meet each obstacle with a sense of acceptance yet determination. His ability to move on inspires family and friends. Even now, Jamie is searching for new opportunities and not willing to let life pass him by.

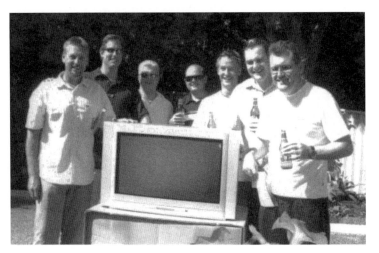

From left to right: Cory, Ado, Morry, Steve, Dean, Stu and Jamie with the TV

Letter from Dr Peter – Joondalup Mental Hospital

Dear Jamie

Thanks for sharing your life story so eloquently and poignantly. I understand a lot more about your spiritual thirst. The sad story of Eva touched my heart.

I was impressed by the detail of your account of your journey and your artistic description of different places in Europe. I am aware that you were "really focused" in the moment while you were travelling. I share your amazement and love for different people from different cultures.

Know that I am often thinking of you and your courage and your inner strength on your current difficult journey.

Dr Peter

Acknowledgements

Jamie would like to thank all his friends and family for their support, over the years and during the development of this book. This includes those times where friends or family were required to assist with his recovery and rehabilitation at locations in Australia and around the world.

Special thanks go to Steve Donaghy, Steve Carroll and Gavin for their help when Jamie was stranded in hospitals in Pamplona and Ireland. The love and support from Eva, Kev, and Aideen was deeply appreciated.

Jamie values all his friends and particularly those that were there for him during his stays in hospital: Stuart and Rose, Ado and Trish, Cory and Tara, Morry and Jo, Anthony and Lucia, Bruce, Ash, Ro and Kate, Trev and Karen, Ryan and Nic, Vaughn and Annie, Anthony and Barbie, Steve (Band) and Pap and Gemma. Thanks also go to Susan and Mark and Rachel, Dean, Steve Duckham.

Those that played (and continue to play) a part in Jamie's rehabilitation also helped greatly. These include Dr Peter, Maree, and the wonderful nurses and doctors at Joondalup and Shenton Park Hospitals.

Jamie asked that family and relatives be given a special mention. The love and support of his family and his relatives helped carry him through the tough times. Jamie recognises the stress that the family has been under and wants to say a special thanks to his Dad, Cam and Maaike (editing) and Andrew for their support and helping to finish the book. And his mum for always being there.

In memory of Eva.

Inner Journey
Learning to live with bipolar

"I'm not crazy I'm just a little unwell.."

Lyrics by Rob Thomas